Adult-Gerontology Acute Care Nurse Practitioner Exam

SECRETS

Study Guide
Your Key to Exam Success

NP Test Review for the
Nurse Practitioner Exam

Dear Future Exam Success Story:

Congratulations on your purchase of our study guide. Our goal in writing our study guide was to cover the content on the test, as well as provide insight into typical test taking mistakes and how to overcome them.

Standardized tests are a key component of being successful, which only increases the importance of doing well in the high-pressure high-stakes environment of test day. How well you do on this test will have a significant impact on your future, and we have the research and practical advice to help you execute on test day.

The product you're reading now is designed to exploit weaknesses in the test itself, and help you avoid the most common errors test takers frequently make.

How to use this study guide

We don't want to waste your time. Our study guide is fast-paced and fluff-free. We suggest going through it a number of times, as repetition is an important part of learning new information and concepts.

First, read through the study guide completely to get a feel for the content and organization. Read the general success strategies first, and then proceed to the content sections. Each tip has been carefully selected for its effectiveness.

Second, read through the study guide again, and take notes in the margins and highlight those sections where you may have a particular weakness.

Finally, bring the manual with you on test day and study it before the exam begins.

Your success is our success

We would be delighted to hear about your success. Send us an email and tell us your story. Thanks for your business and we wish you continued success.

Sincerely,

Mometrix Test Preparation Team

Need more help? Check out our flashcards at: http://MometrixFlashcards.com/NP

TABLE OF CONTENTS

Top 20 Test Taking Tips

1. Carefully follow all the test registration procedures
2. Know the test directions, duration, topics, question types, how many questions
3. Setup a flexible study schedule at least 3-4 weeks before test day
4. Study during the time of day you are most alert, relaxed, and stress free
5. Maximize your learning style; visual learner use visual study aids, auditory learner use auditory study aids
6. Focus on your weakest knowledge base
7. Find a study partner to review with and help clarify questions
8. Practice, practice, practice
9. Get a good night's sleep; don't try to cram the night before the test
10. Eat a well balanced meal
11. Know the exact physical location of the testing site; drive the route to the site prior to test day
12. Bring a set of ear plugs; the testing center could be noisy
13. Wear comfortable, loose fitting, layered clothing to the testing center; prepare for it to be either cold or hot during the test
14. Bring at least 2 current forms of ID to the testing center
15. Arrive to the test early; be prepared to wait and be patient
16. Eliminate the obviously wrong answer choices, then guess the first remaining choice
17. Pace yourself; don't rush, but keep working and move on if you get stuck
18. Maintain a positive attitude even if the test is going poorly
19. Keep your first answer unless you are positive it is wrong
20. Check your work, don't make a careless mistake

Foundations of Practice

ACNP's role as a care provider to high-acuity patients

The acute care nurse practitioner will encounter more high-acuity patients than the nurse practitioner that works in, say, a family medicine clinic. High-acuity patients are patients whose conditions are more critical, less stable, and require more attention; emergency departments, operating rooms, and intensive care units are areas of the hospital that see a high volume of high-acuity patients. The ANA and the AACN have established a set of components that comprise the role of the acute care nurse practitioner when working with high-acuity patients. The ACNP should include the following components in the workup of every high-acuity patient: a comprehensive health history, a comprehensive physical examination, a health risk profile and analysis, a differential diagnosis based on diagnostic reasoning, a therapeutic intervention plan, and consultation with health care providers in other specialties.

Patient history

The patient interview is the first step in the process of treating a patient, and it is often where the most important information is obtained. Because it is such a crucial part of the overall assessment of the patient, it is important to make the patient feel comfortable. You are not likely to get a great deal of information from a patient if you make a negative impression. If possible, conduct the interview in a quiet area. If this is not a possibility, remain calm and relaxed as you interview the patient, and take your time both when asking questions and listening to the answers. If you give the patient the impression that you are impatient or in a rush, he or she may become uncomfortable and hesitant to answer questions.

A comprehensive patient history contains numerous components to help the clinician formulate a diagnosis and treatment plan. Demographic information is an important part of the history, and includes information about the patient's age, sex, and race. The source of the patient referral is also included in the history; it is important to know whether the patient was referred by a primary care physician, a cardiologist, or some other doctor. If someone other than the patient is providing the history, his or her name should be recorded. The chief complaint, or the reason that the patient is being seen, is also important to note, along with a detailed history of the complaint, including when the patient first noticed symptoms, if the symptoms are better or worse at certain times, and what the characteristics of the illness are. Any past medical problems and surgeries are documented as well, including diseases and surgical procedures within the patient's family. Allergies, current medications, and social factors/practices are included in the history.

When the clinician is asking the patient about his or her past medical history, it is important that the clinician includes questions regarding screening tests that the patient may or may not have had recently. If the patient has not had appropriate screening, the clinician should investigate and consider ordering any tests that relate to the patient's current condition. Screening tests such as cholesterol, hemoglobin, and serum glucose are routine blood tests and can be done easily. Urinalysis is another simple screening test, as is a blood pressure reading. More involved and time-consuming tests can be ordered for patients when indicated, including sigmoidoscopy and stool guaiac for routine colon cancer screening, Papanicolaou smear for cervical dysplasia and cancer, mammogram for breast cancer, and ECG for heart abnormalities.

Data gathering

The gathering and recording of data are of utmost importance to the diagnostic evaluation process. The history and physical section of the patient chart contains a wealth of information (ideally), and should always be taken into consideration when developing a care plan for the patient. Because any number of clinicians can add information to the patient chart (and because all of these clinicians will be reading this information), it is important to record all information clearly and in an organized manner. This can be a daunting task when you consider all of the different sources of information, including the patient interview, family member interviews, previous charts, and lab results. By keeping this information clear and concise, you can minimize error, and you can be sure that the differential diagnosis is comprehensive.

Data evaluation

The data that are available on the patient chart are an integral part of the patient's overall care plan. However, errors may be present in the records, and these errors may negatively influence clinical decision making; thus it is important to look at the information as a whole. Does it make sense? Make sure that the patient's verbal history agrees with what you see in his or her records. Also, remember that not every test result you see in the patient's chart is necessarily accurate. If a test result doesn't make sense in the clinical picture as a whole, consider why this might be. It could simply be an error (e.g., the wrong number was recorded, the blood was drawn incorrectly), or the patient may have a result that would be considered "abnormal," though for this particular patient it is not. For example, a marathon runner may have a resting heart rate of 40 bpm; while this is a bradycardic rate, it is not pathological, but rather a result of physical conditioning.

Predictive values

Predictive values are of importance to the clinician because although sensitivity and specificity are used to evaluate the effectiveness of a diagnostic test, they are not particularly clinically relevant. Since a patient's disease state is more or less unknown at admission, these parameters are of no help. This is where the positive predictive value (PPV) and negative predictive value (NPV) of a test come in. If your patient tests positive for syphilis, what are the chances that the patient actually has syphilis? The chance that this result is correct is the PPV; this is calculated by dividing the number of true positive results by the number of total positive results (true and false positives). NPV, then, is the probability that a patient with a negative result really does not have syphilis. Dividing the number of true negatives by the number of total negatives will give you the NPV.

Diagnostic testing

Some degree of error is inherent in almost all diagnostic testing. When you order a diagnostic test for a patient, how confident should you be that the result will be accurate? The terms sensitivity and specificity are used to illustrate the accuracy of diagnostic tests. The sensitivity of a test refers to its ability to correctly identify patients who do have the disease. If a test is administered to 100 patients with diabetes, and all 100 patients test positive, the test is considered to have a sensitivity of 100%. If only 85 of those tested have a positive result, however, that means that the test has a false-negative rate of 15%, and a sensitivity of 85%. On the other hand, the specificity of a diagnostic test refers to its ability to identify patients who do not have the disease. If 100 nondiabetic patients are tested for diabetes, and 50 of them have a positive result, the test has a specificity of only 50%.

Differential diagnosis

The differential diagnosis is an important tool that allows the clinician to familiarize him or herself with the patient's condition, understand the condition, create an effective treatment plan, and follow the progress of the patient. To start, thoroughly examine the patient's chart, making a list of all of the abnormal test results and laboratory values. Add to this list all of the patient's complaints. Once this list is complete, organize the test results, labs, and complaints by anatomic location or organ system. After breaking the list down by organ site, look for any relationships between symptoms and/or results. Create another list of those data that seem to be related, and list all of the diseases or conditions that explain the findings, eliminating any that do not fit.

Asking questions to get the most accurate information

Remember, the main goal of the interview is to get the most information you can, and to make sure that the information is accurate. Asking the patient open-ended questions allows for them to elaborate on their symptoms. Only ask one question at a time, so that the patient knows what question to respond to. Be sure to ask questions clearly, and do not use medical terms that could confuse the patient. After you have finished your questioning, you can repeat your notes back to the patient to make sure that you have accurately understood and recorded their complaints. If the patient has anything to add to the account, record that information as well.

Medical reasoning, diagnostic reasoning, therapeutic reasoning, and therapeutic uncertainty

Medical reasoning refers to the process by which clinicians gather data and information about a patient, and, using those data, arrive at a diagnosis and treatment plan. Diagnostic reasoning and therapeutic reasoning are subsets of medical reasoning; diagnostic reasoning is the information that is used to determine the most likely diagnosis, while therapeutic reasoning is the information used to determine what the best treatment is for that particular patient suffering from that particular disease. While the patient is undergoing treatment, it is necessary for the clinician to evaluate the patient's response to treatment on a regular basis. If it is not clear whether the patient is improving, or whether another treatment might be more beneficial, a degree of therapeutic uncertainty is introduced. There is also therapeutic uncertainty when the clinician is trying to decide which treatment option to use if the first treatment fails.

Cultural awareness assessment tool

The cultural awareness assessment tool was developed as a way for APRNs and other health care workers to gauge their own cultural awareness and sensitivity. The assessment tool is a 17-question quiz in which APRNs ask themselves questions about cultural awareness. The

APRN has the option of answering "always," "sometimes," or "never"; 3 points are received for each "always," 2 for each "sometimes," and 1 for each "never." The higher the APRN's score on the assessment tool, the greater his or her level of cultural awareness. Examples of statements included on the assessment tool include "I recognize the cultural differences between members of the same culture," "I have a high level of knowledge about the beliefs and customs of at least 2 different cultures," and "I know the limits of my communication skills with patients from other cultures."

Giger and Davidhizar cultural assessment model

Giger and Davidhizar developed a cultural assessment model to provide the APRN with a framework for assessing culturally diverse patients. The components of the model are as follows:
1. Communication: It is very important that the APRN determine the patient's preferred method of communication, as well as the patient's style of communication.
2. Space: Different cultures have different ideas about how much space is appropriate; it is important that the nurse understand the patient's spatial boundaries.
3. Social organization: Familial organization and responsibility differs between cultures.
4. Time: This is another variable that differs greatly between cultural groups. The APRN should understand that the patient may have a different concept of timing.
5. Environmental control: An individual's spiritual (and cultural) beliefs greatly affect the amount of control a patient feels he or she has over a situation and its outcome.
6. Biological variations: Some illnesses are more common in certain cultural groups than in others.

Resources that are available for the APRN to increase his or her cultural knowledge

Even the most prepared, educated APRN may at some point be required to treat a patient who belongs to a cultural group about which the APRN has little to no knowledge. In these cases, the APRN should seek to learn as much as possible about the culture in an effort to provide the patient with the best possible care. There are various resources available to the APRN who wishes to expand his or her cultural knowledge base. Journals include the International Journal of Nursing Studies, the International Nursing Review, the Journal of Cultural Diversity, and the Journal of Multicultural Nursing. Internet resources include Ethnomed (http://www.ethnomed.org) and the Foundation of Nursing Studies (http://www.fons.org), as well as information on cross-cultural healthcare (http://www.diversityrx.org).

Outcomes management initiative

Ellwood, in outlining the process for outcomes management, compiled a list of what are considered to be the 4 key components of any outcomes management initiative. The first of these components is that the outcomes management initiative should place emphasis on the formation or selection of standards that the clinicians can follow when planning interventions. The second component is that patient function should be measured, along with patient well-being, using disease-specific clinical outcomes as a gauge of progression. The third component is that clinical data and outcome data should be pooled together for others to use as a reference. The fourth component is that the information database should be analyzed by appropriate clinical decision makers.

Clinical prevention

Clinical prevention refers to the practice of maintaining health and wellness and performing tasks that identify risk of disease at an early stage. Clinical prevention may involve screening for risk factors for certain illnesses. If risks are identified as a result, then further steps can be taken to manage these risks and possibly prevent the disease or illness from occurring. Examples of screenings that may be used as clinical prevention include screening colonoscopies, blood pressure screenings, or skin testing. Clinical prevention may also refer to activities that stop a condition from developing. Examples include child and adult immunizations or counseling to teach patients about practicing healthy behaviors. Clinical prevention services may be available through a variety of measures. In hospital settings, some preventive measures are performed as ordered by physicians but many are part of routine nursing practice. Alternatively, some preventive services are available in the community, allowing quick and easy access for the population to receive screenings.

Prevention intervention

Interventions for prevention of certain diseases involve screening and various other practices to determine the level of risk. Screening practices may involve performing lab tests, measuring vital signs, or performing clinical procedures. An example of a screening test would be a blood test to check glucose levels among a group of people. Those with elevated levels may be at higher risk of insulin resistance. Further testing is required on those who showed elevated results. Some prevention measures involve giving medications that will prevent disease development. For example, administering the flu shot to a segment of the population can help to reduce the risk of influenza in the community. Evaluation of effectiveness of prevention measures is important to determine success. Follow-up with patient groups after screenings can determine if high-risk patients developed the diseases they were screened for. Community-wide regimens require tracking of cases through public health records. Follow-up, tracking, and recordkeeping are essential for adequate evaluation of effectiveness of interventions.

Coronary artery syndromes

Impairment of blood flow through the coronary arteries leads to ischemia of the cardiac muscle and angina pectoris, pain that may occur in the sternum, chest, neck, arms (especially the left) or back. The pain frequently occurs with crushing pain substernally, radiating down the left arm or both arms although this type of pain is more common in males than females, whose symptoms may appear less acute and include nausea, shortness of breath, and fatigue. Elderly or diabetic patients may also have pain in arms, no pain at all (*silent ischemia),* or weakness and numbness in arms. Stable angina episodes usually last for <5 minutes and are fairly predictable exercise-induced episodes caused by atherosclerotic lesions blocking >75% of the lumen of the effected coronary artery. Precipitating events include exercise, decrease in environmental temperature, heavy eating, strong emotions (such as fright or anger), or exertion, including coitus. Stable angina episodes usually resolve in less than 5 minutes by decreasing activity level and administering sublingual nitroglycerin.

Coronary artery syndromes

Unstable angina (also known as preinfarction or crescendo angina) is a progression of coronary artery disease and occurs when there is a change in the pattern of stable angina. The pain may increase, may not respond to a single nitroglycerin, and may persist for >5 minutes. Usually pain is more frequent, lasts longer, and may occur at rest. Unstable angina may indicate rupture of an atherosclerotic plaque and the beginning of thrombus formation so it should always be treated as a medical emergency as it may indicate a myocardial infarction.

Variant angina (also known as Prinzmetal's angina) results from spasms of the coronary arteries, can be associated with or without atherosclerotic plaques, and is often related to smoking, alcohol, or illicit stimulants. Elevation of ST segments usually occurs with variant angina. Variant angina frequently occurs cyclically at the same time each day and often while the person is at rest. Nitroglycerin or calcium channel blockers are used for treatment.

Myocardial infarctions

Myocardial infarctions are classified according to their location and the extent of injury. Transmural myocardial infarction involves the full thickness of the heart (the endocardium, myocardium, and epicardium), often producing a series of Q waves on ECG. An MI most frequently damages the left ventricle and the septum, but the right ventricle may be damaged, depending upon the damaged area:
- Anterior wall infarction occurs with occlusion in the proximal left anterior descending artery, and may damage the left ventricle.
- Left lateral wall infarction occurs with occlusion of the circumflex coronary artery, often causing damage to anterior wall as well.
- Inferior wall infarction occurs with occlusion of the right coronary artery and causes conduction malfunctions.
- Right ventricular infarction occurs with occlusion of the proximal section of the right coronary artery and damages the right ventricle and the inferior wall.
- Posterior wall infarction occurs with occlusion in the right coronary artery or circumflex artery and may be difficult to diagnose.

Clinical manifestations of myocardial infarction

Clinical manifestations of myocardial infarction may vary considerably, with males having the more "classic" symptom of sudden onset of crushing chest pain and females and those under 55 presenting with atypical symptoms. Diabetic patients may have reduced sensation of pain because of neuropathy and may complain primarily of weakness. Elderly patients may also have neuropathic changes that reduce sensation of pain. More than half of all patients present with acute MIs with no prior symptoms of cardiovascular disease. Symptoms may include:
- Angina with pain in chest that may radiate to neck or arms.
- Palpitations.
- Hypertension or hypotension
- ECG changes (ST segment and T-wave changes, tachycardia, bradycardia, and dysrhythmias).

- Dyspnea.
- Pulmonary edema, dependent edema
- Nausea and vomiting.
- Decreased urinary output.
- Pallor, skin cold and clammy, diaphoresis.
- Neurological/psychological disturbances: anxiety, light-headed, headache, visual abnormalities, slurred speech, and fear.

Myocardial infarctions currently classified as Q-wave or non-Q-wave:

Q-wave	Non-Q-wave
- Characterized by series of abnormal Q waves (wider and deeper) on ECG, especially in the early AM (related to adrenergic activity). - Infarction is usually prolonged and results in necrosis. - Coronary occlusion is complete in 80-90%. - Q-wave MI is often, but not always, transmural. - Peak CK levels occur in about 27 hours. - Mortality rates are about 10%.	- Characterized by changes in ST-T wave with ST depression (usually reversible within a few days). - Usually reperfusion occurs spontaneously, so infarct size is smaller. Contraction necrosis related to reperfusion is common. - Non-Q-wave MI is usually non-transmural. - Coronary occlusion is complete in only 20-30%. - Peak CK levels occur in 12-13 hours. - Mortality rates are about 2-3%.

Ventricular hypertrophy

Longstanding primary hypertension will eventually take a toll on other organs in the body, perhaps the heart most of all. Left ventricular hypertrophy is the most common complication of longstanding primary hypertension involving the heart. Left ventricular hypertrophy (LVH) is a thickening of the muscular wall (myocardium) of the left ventricle in response to increased pressure in the aorta, as well as increased peripheral vascular resistance. The high pressure in the aorta and other arteries means that the left ventricle must pump harder to overcome that resistance and move the blood into the arteries; the higher the blood pressure, and the longer the pressure is elevated, the harder the left ventricle will have to work, and the thicker the myocardium will become.

Aortic stenosis

Aortic stenosis is a stricture (narrowing) of the aortic valve that controls the flow of blood from the left ventricle, causing the left ventricular wall to thicken as it increases pressure to overcome the valvular resistance, increasing afterload, and increasing the need for blood supply from the coronary arteries. This condition may result from a birth defect or childhood rheumatic fever and tends to worsen over the years as the heart grows.

Symptoms	Treatment
• Chest pain on exertion and intolerance of exercise. • Heart murmur. • Hypotension on exertion may be associated with sudden fainting. • Sudden death can occur. • Tachycardia with faint pulse. • Poor appetite. • Increased risk for bacterial endocarditis and coronary insufficiency. • Increases mitral regurgitation and secondary pulmonary hypertension.	• Balloon valvuloplasty to dilate valve non-surgically. • Surgical repair of valve or replacement of valve, depending upon the extent of stricture.

Peripheral arterial and venous insufficiency

Characteristics that distinguish arterial from venous insufficiency:

Characteristic	Arterial	Venous
Type of pain	Ranges from intermittent claudication to severe constant.	Aching and cramping.
Pulses	Weak or absent.	Present.
Skin of extremity	Rubor on dependency but pallor of foot on elevation. Skin pale, shiny, and cool with loss of hair on toes and foot. Nails thick and ridged.	Brownish discoloration around ankles and anterior tibial area.
Ulcers	Pain, deep, circular, often necrotic ulcers on toe tips, toe webs, heels, or other pressure areas.	Varying degrees of pain in superficial, ir-regular ulcers on me-dial or lateral malleo-lus and sometimes the anterior tibial area.
Extremity edema	Minimal.	Moderate to severe.

Papillary muscle rupture

The atrioventricular valves separate the atria from the ventricles with the tricuspid valve on the right and the bicuspid (mitral) valve on the left. The *papillary muscles* are located on the sides of ventricular walls and connect to the valves with fibrous bands called chordae tendineae. During systole, the papillary muscles contract, tightening the chordae tendineae and closing the valves. One complication of an MI is papillary muscle rupture, usually on the left affecting the mitral valve, with the posteromedial papillary muscle more often affected than the anterolateral. Dysfunction of the papillary muscles occurs in about 40% of those with a posterior septal infarction, but rupture can occur with infarction of the inferior wall or an anterolateral MI. Rupture on the right side results in tricuspid regurgitation and right ventricular failure while rupture on the left side leads to mitral regurgitation with resultant pulmonary edema and cardiogenic shock. Early identification and surgical repair is critical.

Hypertrophic cardiomyopathy

Hypertrophic cardiomyopathy (also known as asymmetric septal hypertrophy) is a rare genetic and occasionally idiopathic disorder that is often undetected until adolescence when the increasing symptoms become noticeable. With hypertrophic cardiomyopathy, the heart mass and size increase, especially with thickness along the septum, resulting in smaller ventricular capacity so that the ventricles fill less efficiently and the atria have to work harder. This thickening may be asymmetrical. The disease may be nonobstructive or obstructive. The increased size of the septum may pull structures, such as the mitral valve, out of alignment, causing some obstruction of the flow of blood through the valve to the aorta (idiopathic hypertrophic subaortic stenosis). The changes in the ventricles may result in increasing diastolic abnormalities although systolic function is usually normal or high. When diagnosed in young people, the disease is often more severe than in those who are diagnosed later in life.

Vasculitis

Vasculitis is a syndrome in which the walls of the blood vessels become inflamed, causing a disruption of blood flow and resulting in either transient or prolonged ischemia. The most common vasculitis is giant-cell arteritis (GCA) (sometimes called temporal arteritis, because the temporal artery is commonly, but not uniquely, involved); the disease is characterized by a mononuclear infiltrate of lymphocytes and plasma cells that form into giant cells containing multiple nuclei. Large- and medium-sized arteries are affected by GCA. Polyarteritis nodosa (PAN), on the other hand, involves medium and small arteries, and is characterized by an infiltrate of neutrophils. The neutrophils degranulate, causing focal, segmental necrosis of the vessels and surrounding tissue. Henoch-Schönlein purpura is also a necrotizing vasculitis similar to PAN, though it occurs mostly in children, and is limited to the skin, small and large bowel, and kidneys.

Hypovolemic shock

Hypovolemic shock occurs when there is inadequate intravascular fluid.
- The loss may be *absolute* because of an internal shifting of fluid or an external loss of fluid, as occurs with massive hemorrhage, thermal injuries, severe vomiting or diarrhea, and injuries (such as ruptured spleen or dissecting arteries) that interfere with intravascular integrity.
- Hypovolemia may also be *relative* and related to vasodilation, increased capillary membrane permeability from sepsis or injuries, and decreased colloidal osmotic pressure that may occur with loss of sodium and some disorders, such as hypopituitarism and cirrhosis.

Hypovolemic shock is classified according to the degree of fluid loss:
- Class I: <750 ml or ≤15% of total circulating volume (TCV).
- Class II: 750-100 ml or 15-30% of TCV.

- Class III: 1500-2000 ml or 30-40% of TCV.
- Class IV: >2000 ml or >40% of TCV.

Pneumonia

Pneumonia, when it presents in a young, otherwise healthy adult, has a pretty standard presentation, and is not a terribly complicated diagnosis to make. The patient with pneumonia will be febrile and diaphoretic, and will complain of chills, fatigue, and difficulty breathing. The patient will produce sputum while coughing, and the sputum may be bloody. Chest pain, headache, and body aches are also common complaints. In the older patient, however, many of these symptoms may be either blunted or absent. The individual may complain of a general, nonspecific ill feeling (malaise), along with loss of appetite and weight loss. Confusion may also result because of a lack of cerebral perfusion. Tachypnea and tachycardia are common. The patient may or may not be febrile, and may or may not have a productive cough.

Interstitial lung disease

Interstitial lung disease (ILD) is actually a group of diseases characterized by a thickening of the alveoli and the tissue surrounding the alveoli (the interstitium). The thickening of the lung tissue is caused by inflammation and subsequent scarring and fibrosis; in some cases, the cause is known (e.g., sarcoidosis, asbestosis) and in others it is not (so-called idiopathic pulmonary fibrosis). ILD is a progressive disease; there is no absolute cure for the disease. Patients are treated with corticosteroids, which reduce the inflammation and swelling (due to the accumulation of fluid, or edema) of the interstitium. Immunosuppressive drugs may also be beneficial by helping to quell the inflammatory response. Drugs known as angiofibrotics are used to treat patients with ILD as well; these drugs can help slow the process of fibrosis, though they cannot reverse the damage that has already occurred. Patients with severe alveolar noncompliance and subsequent hypoxemia may require oxygen therapy, though this leads to further lung damage over time.

Acute respiratory distress syndrome

Acute lung injury (ALI) comprises a syndrome of respiratory distress culminating in acute respiratory distress syndrome (ARDS). ARDS is damage to the vascular endothelium and an increase in the permeability of the alveolar-capillary membrane when damage to the lung results in toxic substances (gastric fluids, bacteria, chemicals, or toxins emitted by neutrophils as part of the inflammatory-mediated response) reducing surfactant and causing pulmonary edema as the alveoli fill with blood and protein-rich fluid and collapse. Atelectasis with hyperinflation and areas of normal tissue occur as the lungs "stiffen." The fluid in the alveoli becomes a medium for infection. Because there is neither adequate ventilation nor perfusion, the result is increasing hypoxemia and tachypnea as the body tries to compensate to maintain a normal $paCO_2$. Symptoms are characterized by respiratory distress within 72 hours of surgery or a serious injury to a person with otherwise normal lungs and no cardiac disorder. Untreated, the condition results in respiratory failure, multi-organ failure, and a mortality rate of 5-30%.

Airflow obstruction

The 5 mechanisms by which airflow can be compromised and/or obstructed include expiratory airway collapse, bronchospasm, mucosal inflammation and edema, mucinous gland hypertrophy, and external compression of the airway. Expiratory airway collapse occurs in patients with loss of rigidity of the cartilage backbone of the airways. As air is forced out of the airways during expiration, the softened cartilage can no longer hold the airways open, and they collapse in on themselves. Symptoms of expiratory airway collapse mimic asthma and chronic obstructive pulmonary disease (COPD), but although they may have similar presentations, the mechanisms are different. The softening of cartilage that leads to expiratory airway collapse is called tracheobronchomalacia. Expiratory airway collapse can also be caused by excessive dynamic airway collapse (EDAC), which is due not to softening of the cartilage but rather a bulging of the airway membrane into the lumen during expiration.

Bronchospasm is a mechanism of airway obstruction occurring when histamine is released from mast cells (in response to an allergy, irritant, or drug), causing a constriction of the muscular walls of the bronchioles. Mucosal inflammation and edema is fairly self-explanatory as a mechanism of airway obstruction; inflammatory cells accumulate in the mucosa (due to mucosal irritation), resulting in an increase in vascular permeability, and subsequent edema (swelling). This mechanism is seen in patients with COPD (a disease complex that includes chronic bronchitis and emphysema). Mucinous gland hypertrophy is a result of chronic stimulation of the glands (also seen in COPD); the glands increase in size, obstructing the airway lumen. External compression of the airway is also fairly self-explanatory; this is typically due to presence of a tumor pressing on the airway.

Respiratory system changes

As a patient ages, the respiratory system changes in the following ways:
- Rib cage more rigid – There will be more width measured across the anteroposterior chest. When a patient gets old, there aren't as many alveoli. They get inflexible and can no longer draw back. This means that the patient cannot breathe out as well, leading to more residual volume. There is less basilar inflation and the patient cannot get foreign bodies out as well. This condition also happens to someone who has kyphosis.
- Lessened ability for the chest wall to work so that it is harder to take a deep inhalation.
- Trachea and bronchi get bigger in measurement so that there is more unused area and lessened air volume that gets to the alveoli. Small airway shutting means there is less vital capacity and more residual volume.
- Lung parenchyma is not as elastic so that the alveoli do not work as well.
- Breaths are not as deep; coughs are not as forceful because the muscles are not as strong.

Tuberculosis

Currently, the Centers for Disease Control and Prevention (CDC) recommends a 4-drug regimen for the treatment of tuberculosis. These 4 drugs are isoniazid, rifampin, pyrazinamide, and ethambutol. The regimen calls for the 4 drugs to be taken together for 8 weeks; pyrazinamide and ethambutol are then discontinued while the patient continues to take isoniazid and rifampin for the remaining 4 months. Two major problems exist regarding this treatment regimen: patient compliance and drug resistance. Patient noncompliance is common because of the nature of the side effects of the drugs. Most of these drugs, rifampin especially, have side effects that are not well tolerated by the patient. Isoniazid, rifampin, and pyrazinamide are each known to cause hepatitis; when the 3 are taken together, the risk of hepatitis increases, as do the side effects associated with hepatotoxicity. The other major problem associated with tuberculosis treatment is drug resistance; typically, drug regimens for tuberculosis only work for a period of time before the disease becomes resistant to the drugs.

Chronic diarrhea

Chronic diarrhea is more than three bowel movements per day, with watery stools lasting more than two weeks. It is more common and potentially more serious for babies and elders. The most common cause is infectious, but chronic diarrhea in the elderly can also be caused by inflammatory bowel disease, diverticulitis, colon cancer, medication side effects, and irritable bowel syndrome. Take a careful history, including a list of travel destinations. Look for these signs and symptoms of dehydration in the Physical Exam: Flushed, dry skin; dark, scanty urine; fast pulse and respiration; fever; vomiting or nausea; head rushes; thirst; dry mouth; anorexia; chills; tingling; cramps; exhaustion; confusion; seizures; unconsciousness. Send stools to the lab for culture, ova and parasites, occult blood, fecal leukocytes, and *C. difficile* toxin, especially if the patient was recently hospitalized. Collect blood for a CBC and electrolytes. Order abdominal x-ray, and follow up with barium enema or colonoscopy, if indicated. Treat the underlying cause. Significantly dehydrated patients require hospital admission for IV therapy.

Gastroesophageal reflux disease

Gastroesophageal reflux disease (GERD) is a disease in which the mucosal lining of the esophagus is damaged because of reflux of acid from the stomach into the esophagus. The disease causes the symptom known as "heartburn," among other symptoms, and there are a variety of drugs that are used to treat the disease. The first group of drugs is the proton pump inhibitors (PPIs); these drugs alleviate the symptoms of GERD by inhibiting the production of stomach acid. A drug called sucralfate is also used to treat GERD, but by a different mechanism; sucralfate is what is known as a coating agent, meaning that it helps to form a protective layer over the esophageal mucosa. A group of drugs called "promotility" drugs are sort of a last line of defense for individuals who do not respond well to PPIs. Promotility drugs (such as metoclopramide and ondansetron) are typically used as antinausea medications; they tighten the lower esophageal sphincter and promote quicker emptying of the gastric contents.

Gastroesophageal reflux disease (GERD) has several different potential causes:
- Occasional GERD symptoms can be due to consumption of spicy foods or coffee, increased alcohol consumption.
- Viral gastritis may lead to GERD.
- Smoking can increase acid production in the stomach and cause GERD.
- A stressful lifestyle can increase acid production in the stomach.
- A relaxed lower esophageal sphincter also contributes to GERD symptoms.

Patients will complain of burning in the chest or throat with a bad taste in the back of the mouth. They may have a chronic, mild cough from throat irritation. Nausea and vomiting can occur. They may notice that these symptoms are aggravated after meals or when lying down.

Treatment of GERD includes lifestyle modifications with dietary changes, quitting smoking and drinking alcohol, and decreasing daily stress. Avoiding lying down after meals can help. Antacids, H_2-blockers or proton pump inhibitors may be necessary to control the symptoms. Treating GERD symptoms is important to prevent permanent damage to the esophageal mucosa.

Crohn disease and ulcerative colitis

Crohn disease and ulcerative colitis (UC) are often confused with one another. However, there are striking differences between the two. Presentation for both diseases is variable, though diarrhea is very common for both, as is abdominal pain, cramping, and distention. Diarrhea associated with Crohn disease usually occurs a few times a week, usually after meals, and is not remarkable for blood or mucus. UC, on the other hand, is associated with multiple bouts of bloody diarrhea with mucus daily. UC is limited to the colon, while Crohn disease may present anywhere along the alimentary tract, though most cases involve the terminal ileum and cecum. Because only the colon is involved in UC, surgical removal of the colon is considered curative in patients with fulminant disease. Crohn disease, on the other hand, is not considered curative by surgery. The pattern of inflammation in UC is limited to the mucosa, while Crohn disease is more severe, often with transmural (involving the entire thickness of the wall) inflammation.

Ulcerative colitis (UC) is characterized by chronic inflammation of the colon, resulting in deep ulcers that involve the entire wall of the colon (transmural inflammation). Surgical resection of the colon is typically curative of the disease; however, preservation of the colon may be possible by controlling the disease with medication. Aminosalicylates, such as sulfasalazine and mesalazine, have resulted in marked improvement in patients with less severe disease. Steroids, such as prednisone, prednisolone, and hydrocortisone, are also somewhat effective in controlling UC, though the side effects of corticosteroids are somewhat undesirable. In patients with more severe UC, reasonable relief from symptoms may be achieved through low doses of some of the relatively mild chemotherapeutic drugs, including methotrexate, mercaptopurine, and azathioprine. Immunosuppressive therapy with tacrolimus (a drug commonly used to prevent rejection of transplanted solid organs) can also decrease inflammation.

Transient ischemic attack

A transient ischemic attack (TIA), or "mini-stroke," occurs because of atherosclerosis in the brain's arteries. This buildup of cholesterol, or plaque, causes a temporary decrease in oxygen to a certain portion of the brain. About one-third of patients who have a TIA will eventually have a stroke, with most of those occurring within the next year.

Patients will have symptoms similar to a stroke with possible hemiparesis, garbled speech, dizziness, and possible loss of vision in one eye. The difference between a stroke and a TIA is that, with a TIA, the symptoms will resolve spontaneously within 24 hours. There are no residual effects from a TIA.

Patients who have had a TIA should be started on anticoagulant or antiplatelet medications. Low-dose aspirin should be given daily. Medications such as Plavix® or Aggrenox® help to prevent platelet aggregation but do not require routine lab work for monitoring like Coumadin®. Lifestyle changes should be implemented, including eating foods lower in fat and cholesterol, quitting smoking, and losing weight if necessary.

Status epilepticus

Status epilepticus, a condition in which the sufferer is in a persistent state of seizure, has several causes, ranging from alcohol withdrawal to noncompliance in epileptic patients to brain tumor; some of these causes (e.g., brain tumor) do not respond to medication. For others, pharmacologic intervention may help control seizures. Benzodiazepines, especially diazepam and lorazepam, have proven to be very effective in controlling status epilepticus. Before the use of benzodiazepines, the most popular drugs for treating status epilepticus included barbiturates, such as sodium pentothal and pentobarbital, and phenytoin. Phenytoin and sodium pentothal are still used today for patients who are either refractory to or cannot tolerate treatment with benzodiazepines.

Nephrotic syndrome

Nephrotic syndrome is a group of diseases in which the renal capillaries are damaged by inflammation, causing them to become leaky; the damaged capillaries allow for protein and fluids to leak out into the surrounding tissue, causing edema. The causes of nephrotic syndrome are classified as either primary (those that are intrinsic to the kidney, though the exact cause is unknown) or secondary (those that result from other disease processes, such as lupus or diabetes). There is no cure for nephrotic syndrome, and the treatment depends on the cause. For the primary nephrotic syndromes, a diuretic such as furosemide is used to control fluid retention; maintenance of the disease includes monitoring of fluid intake and kidney function. For the secondary nephrotic syndromes, treatment is tailored to the underlying disease; for example, cyclosporin may be used to control autoimmune nephron damage, while diet may help reduce diabetic nephropathy.

Issues that hemodialysis patients face

Patients with end-stage renal disease (ESRD) eventually require hemodialysis, typically when the creatinine clearance is less than 10 mL/min. Hemodialysis is an effective replacement for blood filtration in patients whose kidneys can no longer perform that duty. Even though the hemodialysis patient is carefully monitored before, during, and after dialysis treatments, more than a few complications exist. It is very important that a fluid balance is maintained at all times; many dialysis patients suffer from episodes of hypertension, when too much fluid is filtered and not enough is replaced. Muscle cramps are another common complication, occurring when the patient drinks too much fluid between treatments, necessitating removal of a larger volume of fluid in a short period of time. Not just fluid balance but electrolyte balance is important; an increase or decrease in serum potassium can cause arrhythmias and chest pain during dialysis as well. Circulation of blood through the dialysis machine invariably increases red cell hemolysis, which, over time, can lead to anemia in the dialysis patient.

Type I and type II diabetes

Exercise is important for overall cardiovascular health; lack of exercise has been associated with various health problems, including high blood pressure, atherosclerosis, and type II diabetes. Exercise can be beneficial for diabetic patients, although special precautions must be taken, because there are associated risks as well. Type I diabetics will see an improvement in both cardiovascular function and overall health and well-being; however, exercise can make it more difficult to control blood sugar levels. The type I diabetic should never begin an exercise regimen unless his or her disease is under control. Type I diabetics will also see an improvement in cardiovascular function, in addition to weight loss, which (along with proper diet) may slow or even reverse the diabetic state. The type II diabetic should be evaluated by a practitioner before beginning any exercise plan; ischemia, repetition injury, trauma, and heat exhaustion are among the risks for these patients.

Complications of diabetes mellitus result in increased risk of multiple infections for the diabetic patient. Diabetic patients who suffer from diabetic neuropathy (or peripheral sensory neuropathy) are sometimes unaware of trauma to the distal extremities. Combined with the vascular insufficiency that is common in diabetic patients, poor wound healing ensues. This leaves the diabetic patient susceptible to infection, particularly anaerobic bacterial infections such as Clostridium perfringens, the causative agent of gangrene. Diabetic patients, especially those who do not have their disease under control, often suffer from Candida infections, due to the presence of glucose in the urine. Pseudomonas aeruginosa is a common cause of outer ear infections in diabetic patients. Sinus infection caused by saprophytic fungi (most commonly Rhizopus and Mucor) is also seen; this type of infection is called rhinocerebral mucormycosis.

Diabetes insipidus

Diabetes insipidus (DI) has a much different origin (origins, really) than that of the more well-known diabetes mellitus (DM). Both DI and DM are characterized by an increase in urine production, which may be the most notable, and therefore the presenting, symptom. The urine collected from patients with DI, however, is strikingly different in that, in addition to the low specific gravity, it also has a low osmolality. The dilute urine eliminates DM from the differential. DI, rare as it is, has 4 possible causes. Nephrogenic DI occurs when the kidney's collecting tubules (where the urine is concentrated) become resistant to antidiuretic hormone (ADH). Primary polydipsia occurs when the patient drinks excessive amounts of water, diluting the concentration of ADH. Gestational DI is a result of increased ADH metabolism in pregnant women. The most common cause of DI, however, is trauma in which the pituitary is damaged.

Addison disease

Addison disease occurs when the adrenal cortex functions below baseline. The adrenal cortex is the rim of tissue that surrounds the bulk of adrenal tissue, the medulla. The cortex is responsible for the production of aldosterone, cortisol, and weak androgens. Dysfunction of the cortex can either result from a deficiency intrinsic to the gland (primary adrenal insufficiency) or from impaired secretion of adrenocorticotropic hormone (ACTH) by the pituitary gland (secondary adrenal insufficiency). Addison disease can result through a number of different mechanisms, including destruction of the adrenal cortex by antibodies (autoimmune adrenalitis, the most common cause of Addison), infection (AIDS, tuberculosis [TB]), or adrenal hemorrhage (Waterhouse-Friderichsen syndrome).

Maintenance therapy includes replacement of cortisol (a glucocorticoid that increases the blood glucose level in response to stress) with either hydrocortisone or prednisolone, as well as replacement of aldosterone (a mineralocorticoid responsible for the retention of sodium and water at the distal convoluted tubule) with fludrocortisone. An acute attack of Addison disease, called an Addisonian crisis, is a life-threatening medical emergency, and requires treatment with intravenous cortisone, saline, and glucose.

Hyperthyroidism

Hyperthyroidism is a disease in which the thyroid tissue becomes overfunctional, producing large amounts of triiodothyronine and thyroxine (T3 and T4, respectively); this results in an excess of both of these hormones in the circulation. There are 2 groups of medications that are typically indicated in patients with hyperthyroidism; these medications do not cure the disease, but only control it, and they may lose effectiveness over time. Thyrostatic drugs, such as propylthiouracil, are used to prevent the conversion of thyroxine (which is mostly inactive) into triiodothyronine (the active thyroid hormone). Beta-blockers are also used in conjunction with thyrostatic drugs, though they are used for their palliative effects. An excess of circulating thyroid hormone causes stimulation of the sympathetic nervous system, resulting in anxiety, tremor, and increased heart rate; beta-blockers help to control these symptoms. For patients with disease that is refractory to thyrostatic treatment, radioiodine ablation therapy and surgical removal of the thyroid gland remain as viable treatment options.

Thyroid storm

Thyroid storm (aka thyrotoxic crisis) occurs in hyperthyroid patients when the body is pushed past the threshold of being able to maintain metabolic function through compensation. This is a life-threatening state. Patients presenting with thyroid storm typically are hyperthermic, tachycardic, and in a state of anxiety or agitation. It is important to ask the patient whether he or she has any other existing conditions, and whether or not he or she has been sick lately; this is because thyroid storm is often triggered by acute illness. The defining lab value is a marked increase in free T4 (thyroxine) with a not so marked increase in total T4.

Systemic lupus erythematosus

Systemic lupus erythematosus (SLE) is an autoimmune disease in which the body produces antibodies to its own tissues (especially the kidneys, skin, heart, joints, and blood vessels), causing inflammation and resultant damage to the tissue (which causes a subsequent decrease in the function of the tissue/organ). There is no cure for the disease, and so treatment is aimed at controlling symptoms. Aspirin, ibuprofen, and acetaminophen may be prescribed for pain. Steroids such as prednisone are an integral part of treatment in that they help to reduce inflammation; immunosuppressive and cytotoxic drugs such as cyclophosphamide also help to reduce inflammation by suppressing those cells that produce antibodies. Hydroxychloroquine, an antimalarial drug, has also been shown to improve joint and dermatologic symptoms.

SLE is more common in women than men, and has a peak incidence in the reproductive years. SLE can be a difficult disease to diagnose, because the initial symptoms are often vague and nonspecific. Mild to moderate anemia and an increased erythrocyte sedimentation rate are clues to the disease, but, again, these are nonspecific. Definitive diagnosis is made with a positive antinuclear antibody (ANA) test, along with a constellation of symptoms that include the following: malar rash (a red butterfly-shaped rash across the bridge of the nose and the cheeks); discoid rash (a raised scar-like lesion); photosensitivity; painful ulcers in the nose and mouth; nonspecific arthritis; pericarditis and/or pleuritis (serous inflammation of the pericardial sac and lining of the chest wall); proteinuria due to glomerular basement membrane damage; pancytopenia; antibodies to double-stranded DNA.

Rheumatoid arthritis

Rheumatoid arthritis (RA) is an autoimmune disease causing chronic inflammation of the joints; there is no cure for the disease, and treatment is palliative. Steroids such as prednisone and NSAIDs are used to reduce inflammation in the joints. Methotrexate, a drug with immunosuppressive abilities, is also used to reduce inflammation. Hydroxychloroquine, an antimalarial drug, has been shown to improve the inflammation that is a hallmark of autoimmune diseases, including RA and SLE. Sulfasalazine, which is classified as a disease-modifying anti-rheumatic drug (DMARD), also helps to inhibit the inflammatory process, though the mechanism is unknown. Tumor necrosis factor (TNF) inhibitors halt inflammation by inactivating TNF, a proinflammatory chemical released by lymphocytes.

Hepatitis A and hepatitis B

Hepatitis A: This type of hepatitis is contracted through the fecal-oral route. Symptoms (nausea, vomiting, and fever) typically appear within 30 days of exposure to the virus. Hepatitis A is self-limiting, meaning that it will run its course and will not progress to the chronic stage of infection.

Hepatitis B: This type of hepatitis is transmitted through the blood of an infected individual; though it may also be passed through body fluids that contain blood, including semen, saliva, vaginal fluid, and breast milk. Symptoms, if they appear, will typically present within 12 weeks of infection. Hepatitis B infection may be self-limiting, or it may transform into a chronic infection.

Hepatitis C, hepatitis D, and hepatitis E

Hepatitis C: This type of hepatitis is also passed through blood and body fluids that contain blood; symptoms (nausea, vomiting, fever, abdominal tenderness, jaundice, pruritus) present approximately 7 weeks after infection. About half of all patients infected with hepatitis C will progress to a chronic state.

Hepatitis D: This type of hepatitis cannot infect on its own; it requires simultaneous infection with hepatitis B. The symptoms, progression, and outcome of hepatitis B/D coinfection are similar to infection with hepatitis B alone.

Hepatitis E: Like hepatitis A, this type is also transmitted via the fecal-oral route, and has similar symptoms, though hepatitis E is more likely to progress to fulminant hepatitis.

Treatment for hepatitis C

Hepatitis C is a chronic viral infection of the liver that is transferred through the blood of an infected individual; unlike hepatitis A and hepatitis B, there is no vaccination for hepatitis C. With treatment, the viral load can be eliminated in approximately half of those individuals infected with the disease. The treatment regimen consists of interferon-alpha injections in conjunction with ribavirin, an anti-viral medication. The regimen is extensive, lasting from 24 to 48 weeks; this, combined with the notorious, sometimes debilitating side effects of interferon therapy, adversely affects patient compliance. It is important that the patient follow through with the treatment, and it is also important that the treatment begin as soon as possible; noncompliance and a lag period between infection and treatment both result in an increase in viral load. The greater the viral load, the less likely that the patient will respond well to treatment.

AIDS patients

Clinical category C is for HIV-infected individuals who exhibit conditions that indicate that the patient has progressed to AIDS status; the HIV-positive patient will develop more opportunistic infections as his or her immune system becomes more compromised as a result of decreasing CD4 counts. Conditions that indicate that the patient has progressed to AIDS status include esophageal, tracheal, bronchial, or pulmonary candidiasis; cervical cancer; disseminated fungal infections, including coccidioidomycosis, histoplasmosis, and cryptococcosis; cytomegalovirus infection with widespread involvement; chronic herpes simplex infection; intestinal fungal infections, including cryptosporidiosis and isosporiasis; Kaposi sarcoma; lymphoma; disseminated Mycobacterium infection (tuberculosis, mycobacterium avium intracellulare, Mycobacterium kansasii); pneumocystic pneumonia and other recurrent pneumonias; CNS infections, including toxoplasmosis; HIV wasting syndrome.

Bacterial meningitis

Bacterial meningitis is a very rapidly progressing infection of the membranous coverings of the brain (the meninges), and is highly fatal if untreated. In the United States, the most common causes of bacterial meningitis are Streptococcus pneumoniae and Neisseria meningitidis. S. pneumoniae, also called pneumococcus, requires a 2-week course of antibiotics; penicillin is the first line of defense for pneumococcus. For strains of pneumococcus that are resistant to penicillin, treatment is with ceftriaxone, cefotaxime, and/or vancomycin. N. meningitidis, or meningococcus, requires a week-long course of intravenous penicillin or ampicillin; for penicillin-resistant strains, ceftriaxone or cefotaxime is the treatment of choice. Listeria monocytogenes is a common cause of meningitis among neonates, and is treated with a 3-week course of intravenous gentamicin and ampicillin. Haemophilus influenzae, a common cause among infants, is treated with either ceftriaxone or cefotaxime.

Marfan syndrome

Marfan syndrome is a connective tissue disorder caused by a genetic mutation on chromosome 15, resulting in a defect in the glycoprotein fibrillin. Fibrillin is responsible for extracellular matrix formation, as well as for maintenance of elastin. Individuals with Marfan syndrome have manifestations and complications resulting from a decrease in the tensile strength of the elastic fibers in connective tissue. There are many complications of Marfan syndrome, ranging from nonsevere to life-threatening. Weakening of the connective tissue leads to hernia (inguinal, umbilical, and hiatal), scoliosis, lens dislocation, retinal detachment, mitral valve prolapse, pneumothorax, osteoarthritis, gastrointestinal bleeding, and aortic dissection, aneurysm, and rupture.

Traumatic fracture

In instances of traumatic fracture, the possibility of fat embolism should be considered; this is especially true in fractures involving the long bones (femur, humerus). When the bone is fractured, this allows for some of the fatty marrow contained within the bone to escape. Because the fracture and subsequent trauma to the area surrounding the fracture results in broken vessels, it is possible that the fatty marrow can be introduced into the bloodstream. When this happens, the events are similar to that of a deep venous thrombosis; the fat embolus dislodges from the lumen of the vessel and travels to the lung. When the embolus enters the pulmonary circulation, it eventually blocks blood flow as the caliber of the vessel through which it travels decreases, keeping blood from flowing to the lung tissue. The disruption in blood flow results in inflammation and necrosis of the lung, and eventually pulmonary failure ensues.

Multiple-organ failure syndrome

The multiple-organ failure syndrome is defined as failure of 2 or more organ systems. The syndrome is recognized in patients who have been revived from the shock state, and occurs as a result of the body's natural systemic response to shock. Typically within 2 to 3 days of resuscitation, the systemic response is initiated; the degree of this response (largely inflammatory in nature) is dependent on the severity of the initial injury caused by the shock state. Although this inflammatory response typically resolves on its own within 2 weeks, in some patients a sustained elevated inflammation may be noted. The persistent inflammatory response results in a continued increase in cell production, which leads to a hypermetabolic, acidotic state, and this results in the progressive failure of the organs.

Acid-base disturbances

The four types of acid-base disturbances are respiratory acidosis, respiratory alkalosis, metabolic acidosis, and metabolic alkalosis. Respiratory acidosis occurs when the patient is in a state of hypoventilation; because the patient is not expiring carbon dioxide adequately on exhalation, the excess carbon dioxide accumulates in the blood, decreasing the pH. Respiratory alkalosis, on the other hand, occurs in the hyperventilative state; the blood pH increases because of increased loss of carbon dioxide. Metabolic acidosis results from either an increased loss of bicarbonate (through severe diarrhea, for example, which is commonly seen in children) or an increased production of acid (ketoacidosis). Metabolic alkalosis occurs when the level of bicarbonate in the blood is elevated; this can occur as a result of vomiting, or through excess ingestion of bicarbonate.

Osteoporosis

Osteoporosis is a disease in which the density of bone is decreased, leading to a greater risk of pathologic bone fracture. A daily calcium supplement, taken with a vitamin D supplement, can help to increase the mineral density of the bone. Drugs that inhibit osteoclasts, the cells responsible for bone resorption (breakdown), are effective in preventing further bone loss; these drugs include calcitonin (a hormone naturally produced by the thyroid gland) and the bisphosphonates. The hormone estrogen is known to increase the formation of new bone, thereby increasing bone density, and is another reason that hormone replacement therapy is helpful for postmenopausal women.

Gout

Gout is a metabolic disease in which uric acid crystals form and deposit in and around the joints, causing subsequent painful inflammation. One of the first drugs developed for the treatment of gout was colchicine, a derivative of the autumn crocus plant. Although colchicine has fallen out of favor somewhat, it still may be prescribed for the disease, and the side effects of the treatment should be recognized. Colchicine works by inhibiting both the movement of granulocytes (which are responsible for cell-mediated inflammation) and the deposition of uric acid crystals. Colchicine also has the ability to inhibit mitosis, which results in many of the unpleasant side effects; these include diarrhea, vomiting, kidney failure, and bone marrow damage leading to anemia, leucopenia, and thrombocytopenia.

Acute myelogenous leukemia

Acute myelogenous leukemia (AML) is a cancer of the myeloid stem cell line, and can occur anywhere along the maturation timeline for any of the cells from the myeloid progeny, including red blood cells, platelets, monocytes, and granulocytes. AML is most common in adults older than 65 years of age, although there is an incidence of the disease in the third decade of life, as well as in children younger than 2 years of age. Symptoms develop rapidly, and include fatigue, pallor, easy bruisability, petechial rash, shortness of breath, epistaxis, fever, and weight loss. The majority of these symptoms are attributed to bone marrow involvement of the disease, causing anemia and thrombocytopenia, which reflect in the labs as low hemoglobin, low hematocrit, and low platelet count. White blood cell count is high, and there is a marked hypercellularity in the bone marrow and the peripheral blood due to an increase in the production of immature white blood cells (or nucleated red blood cells or megakaryocytes, depending on the type of AML).

Chronic myelogenous leukemia

Chronic myelogenous leukemia (CML) is a myeloproliferative disorder in which there is an uncontrolled production of mature granulocytes (the white blood cells associated with fighting bacterial, fungal, and parasitic infections) by the bone marrow. The disease is unique in that it is associated with a specific chromosomal abnormality, a translocation of chromosomes 9 and 22. The translocation of these 2 chromosomes results in the formation of a protein called BCR/abl, an active tyrosine kinase protein; this protein is responsible for the uncontrolled production of granulocytes. To stop this overproduction, a drug called imatinib, a tyrosine kinase inhibitor, was developed to target the BCR/abl protein. Imatinib binds to the ATP binding site on the BCR/abl protein and halts the phosphorylation of tyrosine, making it inactive. The drug has proven to be very successful in treating CML.

Brain tumors

The most common type of primary brain tumor is glioblastoma multiforme (WHO grade IV astrocytoma). Meningioma, a benign tumor of the meningeal covering of the brain, is next, followed by low-grade astrocytoma (WHO grade II astrocytoma). Individuals with a higher risk of developing a primary brain tumor include those with neurofibromatosis or tuberous sclerosis, as well as those with a family history of cancer. Patients with a brain tumor typically complain of headache, nausea, and vomiting, as well as a change in personality and progressive neurological deficits. For some patients, seizure is the first symptom of brain tumor. CT scan, MRI, and PET scan are all useful in diagnosing a brain tumor.

Polycystic ovarian syndrome

Polycystic ovarian syndrome (PCOS) is a disease of ovarian dysfunction that occurs when the ovaries are overstimulated by excess luteinizing hormone and insulin, which, in turn, causes the ovaries to produce an excess amount of androgens. Although the cause or causes of PCOS are as yet unclear, there is a strong association between PCOS and insulin resistance. Patients who are insulin resistant (but have no disorder of insulin production) have higher levels of insulin in the blood, which may cause overstimulation of the ovaries. However, not all insulin-resistant women develop PCOS, which suggests there may be some genetic component to the disease. In addition to insulin resistance, PCOS has been linked to frank diabetes mellitus, as well as obesity. Symptoms of PCOS include irregular menstruation or absent periods, infertility (due to anovulation), and depression. Symptoms that result from increased androgens include acne, male-pattern hair loss, and increased body and facial hair.

Benign prostatic hyperplasia

Benign prostatic hyperplasia (BPH) is a common condition in middle-aged and elderly men. It is a noncancerous growth of the prostate caused by an increase in the number of prostatic stromal cells. The proliferation of these stromal cells results in the formation of discrete nodules in the prostate. The nodules are almost always located in the transition zone of the prostate (as opposed to most prostate cancers, which arise in the peripheral zone), which is the area surrounding the prostatic urethra. Due to the location of the nodules, the urethra becomes compressed as they grow, resulting in an increase in frequency of urination, as well as urinary urgency. The urethra may become blocked over time, resulting in bladder distension and infection. Alpha blockers and 5-alpha reductase inhibitors can provide relief from symptoms, but will not stop the progression of nodule growth. A surgical procedure called transurethral resection of the prostate (TURP) can provide relief because it removes the tissue that is compressing the urethra.

Hypogonadism

Male hypogonadism means the testes do not produce sufficient quantities of testosterone. Your patient will be impotent, infertile, and have little or no sex drive. Male hypogonadism can be present at birth from Klinefelter or Kallmann syndromes, and may have micropenis and undescended testicles. Hypogonadism can occur later in life from pituitary or testicular tumors, especially if the man must be castrated (orchiectomy) to slow advancing prostate cancer. Hypogonadism results from aging in 30% of men over the age of 50 as **andropause**. Patients present with beard and body hair loss, decreased muscle mass, osteoporosis, gynecomastia (female pattern breast growth), and complain of erectile dysfunction (ED), emotional lability, fatigue, inability to concentrate, and decreased libido. Patients may also have hot flashes. The diagnosis is made based on the clinical picture and the serum testosterone level. Treatment is testosterone replacement therapy, but it can cause polycythemia. A good serum testosterone target level for seniors is 250 to 1,000 ng/dl.

Endometriosis

Endometriosis is the growth of endometrial tissue outside of the endometrial cavity; it may occur on the serosal surface of the uterus or ovaries, in the abdominal cavity, or even as far away as the lungs and brain (though this is rare). It is a debilitating condition for those patients that suffer from it, and there is no cure for the disease. Medications may help relieve some or all of the symptoms, however. For pain relief, NSAIDs are commonly used; prescription narcotics may be necessary to relieve pain associated with more severe cases. Avoiding estrogens can also control symptoms, as estrogen stimulates the growth of endometrial tissue; progesterone therapy may be indicated as well, as progesterone has the opposite effect of estrogen. Oral contraceptive therapy, taken without the placebo pills, is also effective in treating endometriosis, because it eliminates menstruation. Prevention of ovulation (creating a menopause-like state) can be achieved through use of a gonadotropin-releasing hormone (GnRH) agonist such as leuprolide.

Degenerative joint disease

Degenerative joint disease (DJD), also known as osteoarthritis, is a disease of painful, inflamed joints. The pathological mechanism behind degenerative joint disease is twofold: one, the cartilage that acts as a cushion between bones becomes worn and thin, increasing the friction between the bones, and two, the amount of lubricating fluid inside the joint, called synovial fluid, is decreased, which exacerbates the friction. DJD is classified either as primary, meaning that it is related to the aging process, or secondary, meaning that there is another underlying cause of the disease. Secondary DJD may be caused by obesity, pregnancy, diabetes mellitus, previous injury to the joint, and storage disorders such as Wilson disease and hemochromatosis.

Hearing loss

Approximately 25% of adults over the age of 65 have varying degrees of hearing loss. *Risk factors* for hearing loss include:
- A positive family history.
- Chronic exposure to loud noises, especially if hearing protection was not worn.
- Use of ototoxic drugs, like Gentamicin, NSAIDs, loop diuretics, or cancer chemotherapy.

Hearing loss can be either peripheral or central. Peripheral hearing loss results when the ear canal is obstructed by impacted wax, a foreign object, or damage to the middle or inner ear. Central hearing loss is the result of damage to the portions of the brain that are needed for hearing: Vestibulocochlear nerve, brain stem, contralateral inferior colliculus, superior olivary nucleus, inferior colliculi, ipsilateral medial geniculate nucleus of the thalamus, and primary auditory cortex below the superior temporal gyrus in the temporal lobe.

Pharyngitis

Acute pharyngitis accounts for 40 million visits to healthcare providers in the U.S. annually. It affects all ages and both genders. Incidence increases after age 65. Most patients have 3 to 5 episodes per year. Causes are bacterial and viral. Risk factors include: smoking, exposure to secondhand smoke, HIV, cancer, and immunosuppression. The most common bacterial cause is *Streptococcus pyogenes*. Base your diagnosis on the history and physical exam. Perform a rapid strep test or culture and sensitivity. Bacterial treatment includes analgesics and appropriate antibiotics. Pharyngitis can also be caused by these viruses: Rhinovirus; adenovirus; Epstein-Barr; Influenza A; parainfluenza type 2 or 3; corona; enteroviruses (coxsackie and echo); Herpes simplex type 1 and 2; cytomegalovirus (CMV); and respiratory syncytial virus (RSV). RSV can cause severe disease in the elderly and infants. Viral treatment is rest, oral hydration, salt water gargle, benzocaine lozenges, ice cream, Popsicles, and celecoxib 200 mg once daily. Use amantadine and rimantadine only for Influenza A epidemic, as resistance results.

Muscle atrophy

Sarcopenia describes the process of progressive muscle wasting that is seen in the elderly population. Muscle protein production decreases with increasing age, resulting in a loss of muscle mass, and eventually a loss of physical functional ability. Decreased activity and a lack of exercise contribute to the process of muscle wasting. As sarcopenia progresses, it leads to decreased mobility and puts patients at higher risk for developing other health problems. The process of muscle wasting can be slowed, halted, or reversed with treatment. The most effective treatment is exercise, specifically resistance training. Adequate nutrition, including sufficient amounts of Vitamin B_{12}, protein, and calcium is an important part of the treatment regimen. Use of growth hormone, estrogen or testosterone is controversial. Sarcopenia differs from **cachexia**, which is wasting from a chronic disease.

Obsessive-compulsive disorder

Obsessive-compulsive disorder (OCD) is an anxiety disorder in which the sufferer is overcome by obsessive thoughts and attempts to cancel out or neutralize those thoughts through the performance of compulsive rituals. To be classified as obsessive, the individual must have recurrent, pervasive, intrusive thoughts or impulses that cause anxiety for the individual; these thoughts are not related to real-life problems; the individual tries to suppress the thoughts or replace them with other thoughts or actions; and the individual is aware that the thoughts are a product of his or her mind. A compulsion is a repetitive act that the individual feels compelled to perform in order to neutralize an obsession, with the goal of reducing anxiety associated with that obsession. These compulsions continually disrupt the individual's daily activities.

Anxiety

Although anxiety can be strictly psychiatric in nature, there are various diseases and medical conditions that are known to cause some level of anxiety in afflicted individuals. In the case of certain illnesses, the anxiety may either be caused by the disease, or the anxiety may cause or exacerbate the disease. Anxiety is often associated with tachycardia of both ventricular and supraventricular origin, as well as other cardiovascular conditions, including myocardial infarction, congestive heart failure, and mitral valve prolapse. Endocrine diseases are also commonly related to anxiety, especially hyperthyroidism, hyperparathyroidism, and carcinoid syndrome. Irritable bowel syndrome is closely linked to anxiety, as is peptic ulcer disease. Neurological conditions associated with anxiety include epilepsy and other seizure disorders, Parkinson disease, and essential tremor.

Depression

Like anxiety, depression can be strictly a psychiatric diagnosis, or it may be the result of an underlying medical condition. Individuals suffering from depression are sometimes written off by their physicians and APRNs without further investigation as to the actual cause; it is important that the doctor or APRN really listen to the patient and try to determine the origin of the depression because an underlying cause must be identified. Diseases and conditions that are linked to depression include diabetes, hypothyroidism, Addison disease (adrenal insufficiency), Cushing disease, AIDS, chronic fatigue syndrome, fibromyalgia, infectious mononucleosis, systemic lupus erythematosus, narcolepsy, multiple sclerosis, brain tumor, migraines, and sleep apnea.

Major depressive disorder

An individual suffering from major depressive disorder will present with notably depressed mood, lethargy, and fatigue. He or she may complain of loss of appetite, as well as problems sleeping, which may vary from insomnia to hypersomnia, depending on the individual. Agitation and problems with concentration or the feeling of being in a "mental fog" are common, as well as lack of motivation and lack of interest in activities that once were found to be pleasurable/enjoyable. The patient with major depressive disorder may have a pervasive feeling of worthlessness, and may contemplate suicide. The diagnostic criteria for major depressive disorder include at least 1 month of depression without episodes of mania. Treatment includes selective serotonin reuptake inhibitors (SSRIs), mood stabilizers such as lithium and divalproex sodium, and psychotherapy. For patients with refractory depression, ECT may be an option.

Major depressive episode: characterized by sadness, loneliness, guilt, anxiety, irritability, anger, lethargy, apathy, inability to concentrate, insomnia or hypersomnia, loss of appetite, anhedonia, loss of libido, feelings of worthlessness, and suicidal ideation.

Manic episode: characterized by an increase in energy, insomnia, short attention span, racing thoughts, impulsive behavior (spending sprees, drug/alcohol binges, and promiscuity), irritability, euphoria, and delusions of grandeur.

Hypomanic episode: characterized by increased energy, creative thinking, racing thoughts, and uncontrollable laughter. Symptoms are usually not as severe as mania, and episodes are typically shorter.

Mixed affective episode: characterized by symptoms of both mania and depression simultaneously, causing paranoia, confusion, anxiety or panic, fatigue, restlessness, insomnia, and suicidal ideation.

Bipolar disorder

Bipolar disorder is a mood disorder characterized by separate episodes of *both* mania and depression. There are two forms of bipolar disorder:
- Bipolar I disorder, in which the patient has a history of at least one *manic* episode.
- Bipolar II disorder, in which a patient has recurrent depressive episodes along with *hypomanic*, not manic, episodes.

To qualify as a manic episode, symptoms must last a minimum of four days and lead to difficulties with work or social life. The manic patient initially feels creative, euphoric and energetic. Mania degenerates into feeling invincible and destined for greatness. Gambling, spending sprees and foolish investments are common. The manic patient is hyperactive, sleepless, highly distractible, sometimes combative, and very talkative.

Hypomanic episodes must also last a minimum of four days; however, they do not cause work or social problems. Hypomania just seems like a very good mood to the observer.

Bipolar disorder affects 1% of the population. Men and women are equally affected. Onset is usually between the ages of 15 and 30. Patients present with a history of alternating episode of mania and depression. Manic symptoms include feelings of euphoria, poor judgment, risky behavior, inappropriate spending and hypersexuality. Mania is more common in summer. Symptoms of depression include feelings of sadness or hopelessness, sleep or appetite disturbance, loss of interest in activities, and suicidal ideation. Depression is more common in fall, winter and spring. Cyclothymia is mild bipolar disorder, with hypomania and mild depression. Rapid cycling is four or more mood shifts in one year. Treatment options include mood stabilizers, such as lithium or lamotrigine. Antidepressants may trigger manic episodes and are not usually recommended. Complications include suicide, alcohol and substance abuse, financial, work and social problems.

Schizophrenia

Schizophrenia is a chronic psychiatric disorder characterized by an impaired perception of reality. Schizophrenia affects 1% of the population. Men and women are equally affected. However, men are typically diagnosed in their late teens and twenties with more severe disease, and women are usually diagnosed in their late twenties to forties with a milder form. A family history of schizophrenia is a strong risk factor. Signs and symptoms are delusions, hallucinations, inappropriate speech, and outbursts of bizarre behavior. Patients must have at least two signs or symptoms for a minimum of six months, and they must disrupt activities of daily living. Rule out medical causes. Refer to a psychiatrist for antipsychotics and psychotherapy. Haldol, Seroquel, and Thorazine cause tardive dyskinesia (TD). Risperdal and Zyprexa markedly increase the risk of stroke in seniors with dementia.

Blood alcohol concentration

When an individual has consumed 1 or 2 drinks, his or her blood alcohol concentration is near 0.05%; although the individual may not be visibly intoxicated at this point, his or her judgment is impaired, however slightly. Ingestion of 5 or 6 alcoholic beverages (a blood alcohol concentration of about 0.1%) results in slowed response time and reflexes, and the individual may exhibit slurred speech and clumsiness. At a rate of 10 to 12 drinks, the blood alcohol concentration doubles, and the individual noticeably staggers or even has difficulty walking or standing; he or she may become unintelligible. The individual also exhibits extreme emotional responses, ranging from anger to tearfulness. At 15 to 18 drinks, the individual appears confused, and may be unresponsive (in a stupor). At blood alcohol levels above 0.4%, coma, respiratory depression, cardiac arrhythmias, and death can result. Remember, however, that everyone is different, and some individuals can tolerate alcohol better than others.

Alcohol abuse

Eleven percent of seniors abuse alcohol. More men abuse alcohol than women. *Risk factors:* Family history; starting to drink at a young age; and depression. Seniors' livers cannot metabolize alcohol efficiently; therefore, seniors have a lower alcohol tolerance than younger adults and become impaired more easily. Suspect alcohol abuse if your patient has recurrent falls, confusion, blackouts, pancreatitis, intermittent hypertension, liver disease or gastritis. Ask the CAGE questions:
1. Have you ever felt you ought to cut down on your drinking?
2. Have people annoyed you by criticizing your drinking?
3. Have you ever felt guilty about your drinking?
4. Have you ever had an eye-opener drink first thing in the morning to steady your nerves or get rid of a hangover?

Order a liver panel, CBC and ECG. Supplement the patient's diet with folic acid, thiamine, magnesium and iron daily. Arrange for outpatient therapy or residential detox.

Alcohol withdrawal

The symptoms of alcohol withdrawal range from mild to severe, and which symptoms the patient will experience depends upon how long they have been drinking as well as how much they drink on a regular basis. It is important to be able to recognize these symptoms and get an accurate history from the patient or the patient's family. Mild to moderate symptoms of withdrawal include headache, nausea, tachycardia, an increase in blood pressure, sweating, shaking, vomiting, and loss of appetite. For the chronic, severe alcoholic, more serious symptoms can occur with withdrawal, and the patient should be under medical care. These symptoms include delirium tremens (characterized by disorientation, confusion, hallucinations, hyperthermia, hypertension, and tachycardia), seizure, heart attack, and stroke.

For the relief of mild to moderate withdrawal symptoms, benzodiazepines (particularly diazepam) are commonly used. These drugs have a calming effect on the central nervous system, and may help prevent seizure and delirium tremens. Benzodiazepines should be used for as short a time as possible to prevent the patient from becoming dependent and having to suffer through benzodiazepine withdrawal. Carbamazepine (an anti-seizure medication) may be used in place of a benzodiazepine. Beta-blockers are sometimes administered to control blood pressure and heart rate. Anti-seizure medications and lidocaine are used to help treat delirium tremens and seizure, while antipsychotics (such as haloperidol) are used for patients who are combative, aggressive, and/or psychotic.

Toxicity

The patient suffering from amphetamine toxicity will be hypertensive, hyperthermic, tachycardic, and tachypneic. Mental status may range from agitation to frank toxic psychosis, and the patient will appear hyperactive, hyperalert, and possibly paranoid. Clinical findings include dilated pupils (mydriasis), excessive sweating (diaphoresis), flushing, and hyperactive bowel sounds (borborygmi). Significant lab findings include elevated creatine phosphokinase. Similarly, a cocaine overdose will present with hypertension, tachycardia, and hyperthermia, and the patient will appear agitated and anxious. Paranoia is more common in cocaine overdose, with some patients suffering from hallucinations. Clinical findings are similar to amphetamine overdose, with the addition of seizure and perforated nasal septum (accompanied by epistaxis). An elevated creatine phosphokinase is also seen in cocaine overdose, and electrocardiogram (ECG) abnormalities may be noted.

The patient suffering from an overdose of opioids will present in a hypotensive, hypothermic, bradycardic, bradypneic state. The mental status of an opioid overdose patient can range from lethargy to coma, depending on the severity of the intoxication. The patient will move very slowly (if at all), and exhibit slurred speech. Pupils will be constricted (miosis), and bowel sounds will be diminished or absent. Arterial blood gas values will reflect respiratory acidosis, with an increase in blood carbon dioxide concentration.

Carbamazepine is an anticonvulsant commonly used to treat epilepsy, though it is also used as a mood stabilizer in patients suffering from bipolar disorder. An overdose of carbamazepine will result in a hypotensive, tachycardic, bradypneic, hypothermic patient. The patient will appear lethargic, or may even be comatose. Oddly, an overdose of this drug may result in seizure, as well as hallucinations. The patient may have dilated pupils, and may also suffer from nystagmus. ECG abnormalities related to tachycardia are noted.

Drugs associated with the following smells during a suspected overdose or ingestion

Assessing a patient with suspected drug overdose or toxin ingestion can be very difficult; time is of the essence in determining what was ingested so that the patient can be treated immediately. However, many of these patients are unresponsive and thus unable to communicate what exactly they ingested. Many drugs and toxins will leave clues, however, and some can be recognized by a specific odor. A sweet acetone smell is characteristic of multiple drugs and toxins, including grain alcohol, isopropyl alcohol, trichloroethane, chloroform, paraldehyde, and lacquer. An acetone odor is also strongly associated with patients in diabetic or alcoholic ketoacidosis. A garlic odor may be indicative of thallium, arsenic, selenium, or dimethyl sulfoxide toxicity. A violet smell is associated with turpentine ingestion, while cyanide has a characteristic almond odor, and zinc phosphide smells like raw fish.

Serotonin syndrome

The serotonin syndrome is a group of symptoms that occur as a result of overstimulation of serotonin receptors in the central and peripheral nervous systems; it may also be referred to as serotonin toxicity. The clinical picture for serotonin syndrome includes tachycardia, hypertension, hyperthermia, diaphoresis, shivering, tremor, headache, nausea, diarrhea, agitation, and confusion. A patient suffering from serotonin syndrome may exhibit all of these symptoms, or only a few, depending on the level of stimulation of the serotonin receptors. Patients with severe hyperthermia and shock may become acidotic and progress to rhabdomyolysis, renal failure, and seizure. Drugs that have been implicated in contributing to the serotonin syndrome include MDMA (ecstasy), SSRIs, monoamine oxidase inhibitors (MAOIs), cocaine, amphetamines, LSD, lithium, and even certain antibiotics such as linezolid and erythromycin.

Instances in which a patient should be referred to a mental health specialist

An acute care nurse practitioner is trained to recognize psychological needs in his or her patient, and is often able to provide adequate care for the patient. However, there are certain situations that require the intervention of a mental health specialist, such as a psychiatrist. For example, if the patient is suffering from a complex illness or constellation of illnesses, it may be difficult to evaluate his or her psychological health. If the patient has been receiving treatment, and improvements are not seen, a consultation may also be required. Patients with both mental health issues and substance abuse problems require evaluation and treatment by a mental health specialist, as do patients with illnesses that require behavioral therapy. If the acute care nurse practitioner feels that the patient is at a high risk for committing suicide, further psychiatric care must be provided.

Complementary therapies

Complementary therapies are used as well as conventional medical treatment and should be included if this is what the patient/family wants, empowering the family to take some control. Complementary therapies vary widely and most can easily be incorporated into the plan of care The National Center for Complementary and Alternative Medicine recognizes the following:
- Whole medical systems include medical systems, such as homeopathic, naturopathic medicine, acupuncture, and Chinese herbal medications.
- Mind-body medicine can include support groups, medication, music, art, or dance therapy.
- Biologically-based practices include the use of food, vitamins, or nutrition for healing.
- Manipulative/body-based programs include massage or other types of manipulation, such as chiropractic treatment.
- Energy therapies may be biofield therapies intended to affect the aura (energy field) that some believe surrounds all living things. These therapies include therapeutic touch and Reiki. Bioelectromagnetic-based therapies use a variety of magnetic fields.

Iatrogenic illness

An iatrogenic illness is defined as any illness or symptoms that occur as a result of treatment. Of course, treatment is administered with the intent to make the patient better, not worse, but sometimes treatments do have adverse effects; aging adults are especially at risk of developing an iatrogenic illness. Individuals with multisystem diseases or failures, those who take multiple medications, and those who tend toward atypical disease presentation are especially at risk. The longer a patient remains hospitalized, the more likely he or she is to develop an iatrogenic illness as well. Common iatrogenic illnesses include urinary and fecal incontinence, decubital ulcers (bedsores), muscle wasting, drug reactions, electrolyte imbalance, fluid imbalance, and even heart failure. Nosocomial (hospital-acquired) infections may also be considered iatrogenic; pneumonia and wound infections are common nosocomial infections in the older adult.

Nosocomial infection

A nosocomial infection is an infection that a patient develops during his or her hospital stay; it also may be called a hospital-acquired infection, or a health care–associated infection. For an infection to be considered nosocomial, it must occur 48 hours or more after the patient is admitted to the hospital, to be sure that the patient was not infected prior to admission. An infection may also be considered nosocomial if it develops within 30 days of the patient's discharge from the hospital. Some infections, when introduced to a patient, can spread like wildfire from one patient to another if proper precautions are not taken.

There are 6 known routes of microorganism transmission involved in the spread of infection. The first mode is direct-contact transmission, in which an organism is transferred from an infected individual to a susceptible individual through direct bodily contact. Indirect-contact transmission occurs when an infected individual touches and contaminates an object (phone, sink, glove), and the object transmits the organism to another individual. Common vehicle transmission is similar to indirect-contact transmission, but the organism is transmitted through food, water, or medication. When an infected individual coughs or sneezes, organism-containing droplets can land on another individual, resulting in droplet transmission. Airborne transmission is similar, except that the organisms within the droplets can remain suspended in the air for long periods of time and be inhaled by another individual. A less common mode of transmission in hospitals is vector-borne transmission, in which organisms are transferred to the individual through a carrier such as a mosquito.

Any patient in the hospital can acquire a nosocomial infection, although children, burn victims, post-surgical patients, and the immunocompromised (e.g., oncology patients, HIV-infected patients, post-transplant patients) are at much greater risk. Common bacterial nosocomial infections are caused by Escherichia coli, Proteus mirabilis, Pseudomonas aeruginosa, Klebsiella pneumoniae, Clostridium difficile, Acinetobacter species, and Citrobacter species (all of which are gram-negative), as well as Streptococcus pneumoniae and Staphylococcus aureus (both of which are gram-positive). Fungal agents may also cause nosocomial infection, especially the yeasts Candida albicans and Candida glabrata. Common viral causes of nosocomial infection include respiratory syncytial virus (RSV), rhinovirus, influenza, parainfluenza, and enteroviruses.

Fournier gangrene

Fournier gangrene is a relatively uncommon but serious necrotizing infection of the genital area; it is more common in men than women. Although uncommon among the general population, is not uncommon among patients with diabetes mellitus. It is also more commonly seen in immunosuppressed (patients with HIV, patients undergoing chemotherapy) patients, malnourished patients, and chronic alcoholic patients. The disease is caused typically by an infection of both aerobic and anaerobic organisms, and Clostridium perfringens is often identified. Because of the rapidly fatal progression of the infection, it is important to recognize the signs and begin treatment immediately. Fournier gangrene should be suspected when a red plaque is identified on the genitals; the plaque will quickly become purulent and necrotic-appearing; the tissue surrounding may be crepitant because of gas formation from the anaerobic bacteria.

Reducing the spread of infection among patients

Perhaps the most important guidelines for the prevention of transmission between both patients and health care workers are the Universal Precautions guidelines, which state that every patient should be regarded as potentially infectious with regard to handling anything that could potentially transmit a bloodborne pathogen (such as the HIV virus or hepatitis C virus). This includes the handling of blood, tissue, semen, vaginal secretions, and body cavity fluids (synovial, cerebrospinal, pleural, pericardial, peritoneal, and amniotic). Treating every patient as potentially infectious ensures that the most care is taken to protect all patients. This includes wearing gloves (and changing them between patients), gowns, and other protection as necessary. Disposable items should be used whenever possible, and items that cannot be discarded must be disinfected. Frequent and proper hand washing is also extremely important, and all health care workers should keep nails short and clean, as bacteria can hide under long nails and be transferred to patients.

Wound healing

Immediately after tissue injury (within 5 to 10 minutes), epinephrine, norepinephrine, thromboxane, and prostaglandins are released; these mediators initiate vasoconstriction, which functions to control any hemorrhage in the area. This is followed by endothelial retraction, which exposes collagen on the subendothelium. Platelets attach to the collagen using fibrinogen, and the attached platelets then attract other platelets to form a platelet plug; this process is called platelet adhesion and aggregation. The aggregated platelets, which are now activated, release serotonin, histamine, and platelet-derived growth factor (PDGF) to initiate the coagulation cascade. The end result of the cascade is the activation of thrombin, which serves 2 purposes: to convert fibrinogen to fibrin, and to increase vascular permeability. The increase in permeability allows inflammatory cells to move from the bloodstream into the injured tissue. Neutrophils dominate the inflammatory picture in the early stages, and are later replaced by monocytes and tissue macrophages, which clean up the debris. Vasodilation increases the blood flow to the area to deliver more cells, fluid, and nutrients, and contributes to tissue edema.

The proliferative phase of wound healing begins at the end of the inflammatory phase (there is some overlap), usually within 3 to 5 days after the initial injury. Epithelialization is important; the purpose is to create a new layer of epithelium over the surface of the wound. In simple terms, this is a 2-step process: the epithelial cells proliferate from the edges of the wound and grow toward the center as the clot is dissolved. The epithelial cells secrete enzymes to stimulate the formation of plasmin, which slowly dissolves the clot as the epithelial layer is forming. Under the epithelial surface, fibroblasts are synthesizing and depositing collagen and elastin to restore the tissue to its pre-injured state. New blood vessels are formed during this time (a process called angiogenesis) to deliver enzymes, macrophages, and other nutrients and cells. The blood vessels disappear as the need for them decreases. At the end of this phase, the wound tightens as the cells at the periphery contract.

The maturation phase of wound healing consists mostly of the remodeling of collagen in the wound. Collagen remodeling is a somewhat complex process in which collagen is both removed and synthesized. The removal of old collagen from the wound occurs as a result of various enzymes, including collagenases and matrix metalloproteinases. During this remodeling process, type III collagen is slowly replaced by type I collagen, and proteoglycans replace hyaluronic acid, while water is reabsorbed from the area. This eliminates spaces between collagen fibers, and promotes a more orderly distribution of fibers, thus reducing the size of the scar over time.

Age-related considerations

Because each individual patient is exposed to different stressors that can affect the aging process, it is important to consider that some patients may experience adverse health problems, while other patients of the same age may not be affected. As individuals age, the amount of wear on the body, as well as the chance of pathology, increases; just remember that this does not happen at the same rate for every person. Factors affecting the aging process include proper nutrition (or the lack thereof), level of physical activity, smoking, alcohol consumption, environmental or occupational exposures, and socioeconomic standing. Also, remember that as an individual ages, a disease or problem with one organ or organ system will have a marked effect on other systems, because the body is not able to compensate as it once was. Symptoms may not even be noticeable until other functions begin to decline.

Acute confusion

Acute confusion is a serious problem regarding aging patients, and becomes a greater risk the longer the patient remains in the hospital. The development of acute confusion in the aging patient leads to a greater risk of placement in a long-term care facility, such as hospice care or a nursing home, and also has a fairly high risk of mortality. Certain patients, when admitted, are already considered to be at risk for developing acute confusion; this includes patients older than 80 years of age, those already suffering from dementia, and those with preexisting illnesses and comorbidities. Other factors, occurring during hospitalization, may also contribute, including immobility, certain medications, infections, fluid overload, and electrolyte imbalance.

Pharmacokinetics

Metabolism of drugs involves four steps: Absorption, distribution, metabolism and elimination. All of these steps are affected by the age of the patient because the organs involved degenerate from wear and tear. Absorption of most drugs occurs in the small intestine. Drug absorption in older adults may be delayed or decreased due to decreased blood flow to the small intestine. This could change the blood levels of drugs achieved in the geriatric patient. Distribution of the drug is altered due to a change in body composition. Elderly patients have decreased total body water and lean muscle mass. This relative increase in total body fat may increase the duration of action of lipid-soluble drugs. Most drugs are metabolized by either the liver or the kidneys. Decreased function of these organs lead to delayed metabolism and elimination of certain medications.

Polypharmacy

Polypharmacy is a term used to describe inappropriate use of medications. It occurs when medications are taken that are not indicated, medications that have adverse interactions with one another are taken together, and patients take contraindicated medications. Polypharmacy is a common problem in the geriatric population. Most office visits result in new prescriptions being written and patients may accumulate many different medications in their home. Polypharmacy greatly increases the patient's risk of having an adverse drug reaction. Obtain a detailed drug history at each visit. This should include nonprescription medications, herbs, and ethnic medicines like mercury. Educating patients about the problem of polypharmacy is very important. This can occur in the clinician's office or with a community education program.

Tissue plasminogen activator

Tissue plasminogen activator (tPA) is a thrombolytic agent used to dissolve blood clots before they cause irreversible damage to the heart, brain, or other organs. A blot clot is composed of red blood cells, white blood cells, platelets, and fibrin, among other things; when tPA is administered, it binds to the fibrin in the clot. The binding of tPA to fibrin activates another fibrin-bound protein called plasminogen; plasminogen, in its active form, is called plasmin. Plasmin is a strong enzymatic protease that plays a major role in clot lysis; when it is released from its fibrin-binding sites through the binding of tPA, it then breaks apart the fibrin molecules within the clot, initiating the clot-dissolving process.

Theophylline

Theophylline is an aromatic organic compound called dimethylxanthine, belonging to a group of methylxanthines. The mode of action of the drug is as a broad adenosine receptor antagonist; because it is not specific for a particular adenosine receptor, many of its effects are not intended. Theophylline is used mainly for the treatment of asthma and COPD, and it is very effective at treating these diseases. However, because of its nonspecificity, its levels must be monitored in all patients taking the drug to avoid toxicity. Theophylline works by relaxing the smooth muscle surrounding the bronchioles; increasing the heart rate, heart contractility, and blood pressure; increasing blood flow to the kidneys; and stimulating the respiratory center, which is located in the brainstem.

Levodopa

Levodopa, or L-dopa, is a molecule that is the precursor to dopamine, epinephrine, and norepinephrine; it is widely used as a treatment for Parkinson's disease, a degenerative disease of the central nervous system that results in impaired production of dopamine. L-dopa is termed a "prodrug," which means that it is administered to the patient as an inactive drug; once L-dopa enters the body, it is then metabolized into dopamine, the active form, by dopa decarboxylase. The reason L-dopa is administered instead of the active dopamine is because the L-dopa molecule can cross the blood-brain barrier, whereas the dopamine molecule cannot; giving the patient dopamine, then, would be useless, because the dopamine would reside in the peripheral tissues instead of traveling to the brain, where it is needed. When L-dopa is administered, it crosses the blood-brain barrier into the brain, where it can then be metabolized into dopamine.

L-dopa, though it is the most effective drug (really, the only effective drug) for treatment of Parkinson disease, has a number of unpleasant side effects, including nausea, hair loss, anxiety, confusion, and visual hallucinations. The majority of these side effects can be attributed to the way that L-dopa is metabolized once it enters the body. The ideal situation would be that all of the L-dopa, once administered, would cross the blood-brain barrier into the brain, where it would be metabolized into dopamine. However, although the molecules can cross the barrier, not all of them do. The molecules that do not cross into the brain remain in the peripheral tissues, where they too are metabolized into dopamine. This peripheral dopamine supply causes a number of the adverse effects of the drug. To counteract this effect, a drug known as carbidopa, which prevents peripheral metabolization of L-dopa, is administered simultaneously.

Tamoxifen therapy

Tamoxifen is a drug known as a selective estrogen receptor modulator. It has seen great success in the treatment of breast cancers that are estrogen receptor positive; ER+ tumors require estrogen to grow. When the drug is administered (as a prodrug, in actuality), it is metabolized by the liver; its metabolites then bind to estrogen receptors on the tumor cells so that estrogen cannot bind, which in turn stops the tumor from growing. Tamoxifen is typically an adjuvant therapy, meaning that it is given after the primary therapy (e.g., chemotherapy, radiation) in an effort to prevent recurrence. The drug is also given to patients who are considered to be at risk for developing ER+ breast cancer in an effort to prevent the disease.

Erythropoietin

Erythropoietin (EPO) is a hormone produced by the kidneys (and, to a lesser extent, the liver) that stimulates the production of red blood cells. Because the kidneys produce the majority of the hormone, damage to the kidneys can result in anemia. For this reason, erythropoietin is used therapeutically to treat anemia caused by chronic renal failure. Erythropoietin is also common in treating chemotherapy patients suffering from anemia secondary to bone marrow ablation by chemotherapeutic drugs. Erythropoietin has been used to increase red cell production in patients suffering from anemia of chronic disease, which is a complication of longstanding illnesses such as heart failure, liver failure, and autoimmune diseases.

Zidovudine

Although the components of the drug "cocktail" used to treat individuals with HIV infection and AIDS is hotly contested, and there is no perfect combination of drugs, there is one drug that most will agree should be included in any treatment regimen for the disease, and that is AZT, or zidovudine. AZT is an antiretroviral drug that works by inhibiting the action of an enzyme called reverse transcriptase, which is the enzyme that is necessary to make DNA from RNA. Without being able to form DNA, the virus cannot infect host cells. The downside of AZT is that it does not work forever, as the virus eventually develops resistance to the drug. AZT therapy is particularly effective in preventing the virus from being passed from mother to child, and it is given prophylactically to individuals who may have been exposed to the virus.

Rho(D) immune globulin (human) injection

Rho(D) immune globulin (human) is an immunoglobulin (antibody) injection that contains immunoglobulin G (IgG) antibodies (the only class of antibody that can pass from the mother's blood through the placenta to the fetal circulation) against the D (or RhD) antigen on red blood cells. The purpose of the injection is to prevent the mother from creating antibodies against the blood of her fetus, which may result in hemolytic disease of the newborn (HDN). If the mother is Rh negative, and the fetus is Rh positive, fetal red cells that enter the maternal circulation can cause the mother to produce anti-Rh antibodies; these antibodies can then cross the placenta and destroy the red cells in the fetal circulation, causing anemia, jaundice, kernicterus (bilirubin deposits in the central nervous system), and even death. When a small amount of anti-Rh is injected into the mother, it will bind any circulating fetal cells and destroy them before the mother can produce mass amounts of antibodies.

Tacrolimus

Tacrolimus (sometimes referred to as FK506) is a non-antibiotic macrolide drug used for its immunosuppressive ability. The drug works by binding to the FK506 binding protein; this inhibits the transcription of IL-2 (a cytokine that activates lymphocytes) and blocks the transmission of signals between T cells. By disabling IL-2 transcription and T-cell signaling, tacrolimus greatly compromises the body's immune response. For this reason, the drug is widely used to guard against rejection of transplanted solid organs (e.g., liver, kidney, lungs). Although the drug was developed to prevent post-transplant rejection, it has more recently been used (rather experimentally, however) to treat ulcerative colitis. A topical form of the drug has also shown some promise in the treatment of eczema.

Lithium

Lithium exists as an ion in the form of an alkali metal; combined with other elements to form a lithium salt, it is used as a mood-stabilizing drug for the treatment of both the depressive and (to a greater extent) manic phases of bipolar disorder. Lithium works both by decreasing the amount of circulating norepinephrine (a hormone that increases heart rate, blood glucose levels, and alertness) and increasing production of serotonin. Lithium is somewhat unique in that the therapeutic level of the drug is very close to the toxic level; for this reason, blood lithium levels must be carefully monitored to ensure that the patient is within the therapeutic window. Because lithium causes some degree of dysregulation of both water and sodium, patients taking lithium can become dehydrated. It is important that patients remain hydrated and maintain appropriate sodium intake. In addition to regular monitoring of lithium levels, patients should be monitored for both kidney and thyroid function.

Antihistamines

Antihistamines – May cause problems with sight and walking, causing a fall, as well as fuzzy mental ability and an influence on ability to function, which may cause unforeseen hospital visits or having to go to a nursing home. Also can interfere with other medications or make other medications have worse side effects.

Primary dysmenorrhea – Use nonsteroidal anti-inflammatory analgesics. Physical activities, methods of relaxation, heat, and small amounts of oral contraceptives (OCs) may also help.

Hot flashes – Venlafaxine HCL (Effexor SR), which helps hot flashes (as seen in random-controlled trials). The dosage is 25–150 mg daily. Some patients think nonprescription or natural aids are less dangerous than prescriptions, but they can have adverse outcomes or they may interfere with other medications. Ask the patient about any other medications or natural supplements they may be taking.

Gonococcal infection – The majority of cases of PID for females that are engaging in intercourse are gonococcal infections, and they commonly accompany *Chlamydia* infections. Generally you need to medically manage both at the same time. Use ceftriaxone (Rocephin), 125 mg IM and azithromycin (Zithromax), 1 g PO.

Atropine

Atropine is a drug known as a muscarinic receptor antagonist; the drug works by binding to muscarinic receptors, thus blocking acetylcholine from binding to the muscarinic receptors. Acetylcholine, when bound to muscarinic receptors, is responsible for increasing vagal stimulation of the heart; increased vagal stimulation of the heart, in turn, is responsible for slowing the heart rate. In patients with bradycardia resulting from an atrioventricular (AV) nodal block, atropine may be administered to correct the block. When atropine is administered to patients with an AV block, the drug binds to the muscarinic receptors, blocking the acetylcholine from binding; this results in a decrease in vagal stimulation of the heart, which increases the heart rate.

Vasopressin

Vasopressin, or antidiuretic hormone (ADH), is used in a variety of clinical situations. The synthetic form of vasopressin, called desmopressin, is administered to patients either intravenously, nasally, or orally (in pill form). Desmopressin is most commonly used in the treatment of diabetes insipidus, a disease in which the kidney, because of a lack of vasopressin production, does not concentrate urine at the distal convoluted tubule. This results in frequent, excessive voiding of hypotonic urine. Patients with a decrease in vasopressin production benefit from desmopressin therapy. Desmopressin is also used to treat chronic bedwetting in children, and has been shown to improve clotting in individuals suffering from von Willebrand disease, thrombocytopenia, and mild cases of factor VIII deficiency (hemophilia A).

Anaphylaxis

Anaphylaxis is a severe, systemic hypersensitivity (allergic) reaction that is classified as a type I hypersensitivity. If an individual suffering from an anaphylactic reaction is not treated immediately, death is likely. The systemic symptoms of anaphylaxis (hypotension, difficulty breathing, and angioedema) result from the release of large amounts of histamine from mast cells. When released into the bloodstream, histamine causes the bronchioles to constrict; it also causes vasodilation (relaxation of the blood vessels, resulting in a decrease in blood pressure) and leakage of fluids into the surrounding tissue (resulting in edema and a further decline in blood pressure). When an individual is suffering from an anaphylactic reaction, treatment with epinephrine is the best way to stabilize the patient. Epinephrine is a powerful vasoconstrictor, and an equally powerful bronchodilator; it also increases heart rate and stroke volume to counteract the shock that occurs as a result of the anaphylactic reaction.

Activated charcoal

Activated charcoal (or activated carbon) is used in the treatment of patients with acute poisoning associated with ingestion of a chemical or drug. Syrup of ipecac is another method to rid the body of poison, although it causes the individual to vomit; vomiting of a toxic substance can lead to further damage as the substance exits the body, and it also has no effect on substances that have already entered the intestines. Activated charcoal, on the other hand, works by adsorption, meaning that the toxin attaches to the surface of the charcoal molecules, reducing the potency of the toxins. The charcoal (a fine black powder) is usually administered either orally (by giving the patient a solution to drink) or through a nasogastric tube.

Fibrinolytic infusions

Fibrinolytic infusion is indicated for acute myocardial infarction under these conditions:
- Symptoms of MI, <6-12 hours since onset of symptoms.
- ≥ 1 mm elevation of ST in ≥ 2 contiguous leads.
- No contraindications and no cardiogenic shock.

Fibrinolytic agents should be administered as soon as possible, within 30 minutes is best. All agents convert plasminogen to plasmin, which breaks down fibrin, dissolving clots:
- Streptokinase & anistreplase (1st generation).
- Alteplase or tissue plasminogen activator (tPA) (second generation).
- Reteplase & tenecteplase (3rd generation).

Contraindications
- Present or recent bleeding or history of severe bleeding.
- History of brain attack (<2-6 month) or hemorrhagic brain attack.
- Anticoagulation therapy.
- Acute uncontrolled hypertension.
- Aortic dissection or pericarditis.
- Pregnancy. Intracranial/intraspinal surgery or trauma within 2 months or neoplasm, aneurysm, or AVM.

Opiate abuse and withdrawal symptoms

Opioid analgesic therapy is a widely used method of chronic pain control. The severity of symptoms is dependent on the amount and duration of use. Common side effects of abuse may mimic the flu and include increased respirations, diarrhea, runny nose, sweating, coughing, lacrimation, muscle twitching, and increased temperature and blood pressure. Withdrawal symptoms will overlap with abuse symptoms and become worse. Agitation, anxiety, nausea and vomiting, chronic goose bumps, and dilated pupils are also present.

Overdose is treated with naloxone. Withdrawal symptoms can be eased with methadone.

Morphine withdrawal

Morphine is an opioid drug whose main benefit is pain relief. Because it is such a strong pain reliever, morphine is often used to treat the pain associated with cancer, kidney stones, sickle cell crisis, heart attack, bone fracture, and surgical procedures. Along with its strong pain-relieving ability, however, morphine also carries with it a strong addictive component. Patients using morphine to treat pain often find themselves addicted, even after a short period of time. Individuals who have been taking morphine for long periods of time are much more susceptible to the withdrawal symptoms, as dependence increases over time. Withdrawal symptoms include diarrhea, sweating, restlessness, insomnia, tremor, nausea, vomiting, hot flashes, and bone and muscle pain.

Clozapine

Clozapine is a second-generation antipsychotic drug that is used to treat schizophrenic patients with refractory disease (meaning that the disease does not respond to other treatments). Although the drug has proven to be a great treatment for refractory schizophrenia, its use must be carefully monitored, because it has a potentially life-threatening side effect called agranulocytosis. Agranulocytosis, or a lack of granulocytes in the blood, means that the patient does not have the ability to fight off bacterial infections. This side effect occurs in between 1% and 2% of patients taking clozapine, which is not an insignificant number. For this reason, the FDA requires that patients being treated with the drug submit to mandatory weekly blood testing so that granulocyte levels can be monitored, and the drug can be discontinued if levels begin to drop.

Medications that could make an older patient experience incontinence

Older patient – May get incontinence with the use of hypnotics, sedatives, or antidepressants. The first 2 medications cause sedation and muscles that are more relaxed than usual. This is true for everyone, but an older patient can be more affected due to the effects of aging on the central nervous system. There is more muscle relaxation. Antidepressants give anticholinergic outcomes and can cause sedation as well.

Nitrofurantoin (Macrodantin) – Should not be used when there is a problem with renal ability, when there is not enough antibacterial concentration in the urine, or when there is more of a chance of toxicity. If a patient has an ongoing UTI, consider using this drug for prevention, 100 mg PO, qhs. If the patient is elderly, have no serum or tissue gathering for this medication.

Renal calculi – Handle pain first. Use morphine sulfate, 10 mg SC or meperidine (Demerol). Ibuprofen (Advil) can be used if the pain is just starting. Trimethobenzamide (Tigan) may be utilized after the pain regimen has begun.

Haloperidol

Haloperidol is a first-generation, or typical, antipsychotic drug that is used in the treatment of schizophrenia, acute psychosis, mania, and delirium. A more accurate classification of the drug is as a neuroleptic, meaning that it works by blocking dopamine receptors in the brain, specifically in the limbic system, which includes the hippocampus and controls behavior and emotions. Because haloperidol is such a strong anti-dopaminergic drug, it has untoward side effects related to motor function. These side effects are referred to as extrapyramidal effects, and can be disfiguring and even permanent, depending on the amount and length of treatment. Examples of extrapyramidal side effects include dystonia (abnormal, awkward posturing, muscle cramping and spasms), akathisia (internal restlessness and anxiety), bradykinesia (slow movements), and even akinesia (the physical inability to move).

Artificial insulin

Patients with type I diabetes mellitus are born with a defect in insulin production; these patients, then, rely on insulin injections to control their blood glucose levels because they do not produce the insulin necessary to regulate their blood glucose. There are several different kinds of insulin that may be used to control type I DM, and they are classified based on their speed of action. Rapid-acting insulin starts to work within approximately 10 minutes of injection, and the effects continue for 3 to 4 hours; this type of insulin is particularly effective for the patient in diabetic shock (ketoacidosis). Short-acting insulin takes a little longer to begin working, within 30 minutes, and lasts for 5 to 8 hours. Intermediate-acting begins working in 1 to 3 hours and lasts for approximately 16 to 24 hours; long-acting insulin begins working within 4 to 6 hours, and is active for 24 to 48 hours.

Sedation

Sedation may be used for drug-induced coma to treat traumatic brain injury and increased intracranial pressure. The most commonly used drugs are barbiturates (pentobarbital or thiopental) and sedatives (propofol). Barbiturates depress the reticular activating system in the brain stem, an area controlling body functions, including consciousness. Barbiturates with phenyl serve as anticonvulsants (phenobarbitol) but those with methyl (methohexital) do not. If sulfur is added to the compound to replace some oxygen, the barbiturates have increased lipid solubility (thiopental, methohexital, and thiamylal), making them useful as rapid acting anesthetics. Barbiturates have a number of systemic effects. Blood pressure falls and heart rate increases although cardiac output is usually maintained. With hypovolemia, CHF, and β-adrenergic blockade, there may be peripheral pooling of blood and myocardial depression that causes a pronounced drop in BP and cardiac output. Barbiturates reduce cerebral blood flow and decrease ICP, but cerebral oxygen consumption is also reduced. Barbiturates do not relax muscles or reduce sensation of pain.

Sedation used for drug-induced coma often includes propofol. Propofol is an IV non-opioid hypnotic anesthetic, the most common used for induction. It is also used for maintenance and postoperative sedation. Onset of action is rapid because of high lipid solubility, and propofol has a short distribution half-life and rapid clearance, so recovery is also fast. Propofol is metabolized by the liver as well as extrahepatically through the lungs. Propofol decreases cerebral blood flow, metabolic rate of oxygen consumption and ICP, similarly to thiopental. Propofol causes vasodilation with resultant hypotension, but with bradycardia rather than tachycardia. Tachycardia during induction may indicate metabolic acidosis. Propofol is a respiratory depressant, resulting in apnea after induction and decreased tidal volume, respiratory rate, and hypoxic drive during maintenance. Upper airway reflexes are more reduced than with thiopental and there is less wheezing with induction and intubation, so propofol is often used as sedation for those on mechanical ventilators. Propofol has antiemetic properties as well but does not produce analgesia.

Conscious sedation is used to decrease sensations of pain and awareness caused by a surgical or invasive procedure, such a biopsy, chest tube insertion, fracture repair, and endoscopy. It is also used during presurgical preparations, such as insertion of central lines, catheters, and use of cooling blankets. Conscious sedation uses a combination of analgesia and sedation so that patients can remain responsive and follow verbal cues but have a brief amnesia preventing recall of the procedures. The patient must be monitored carefully, including pulse oximetry, during this type of sedation. The most commonly used drugs include:

- Midazolam (Versed®): This is a short-acting water-soluble sedative, with onset of 1-5 minutes, peaking in 30, and duration usually about 1 hour (but may last up to 6 hours).
- Fentanyl: This is a short-acting opioid with immediate onset, peaking in 10-15 minutes and with duration of about 20-45 minutes.

The fentanyl/midazolam combination provides both sedation and pain control. Conscious sedation usually requires 6 hours fasting prior to administration.

Patients intubated for mechanical ventilation are usually given sedation and/or analgesia initially, but medications should be reduced and given in boluses rather than with continuous IV drip with a goal of stopping sedation as it prolongs ventilation time. Typical sedatives include midazolam, propofol, and lorazepam. Narcotic analgesics include fentanyl and morphine sulfate. Uses of sedation include:

- Controlling agitation and excessive movement that may interfere with ventilation.
- Reduce pain and discomfort associated with ventilation.
- Control respiratory distress.

Triglyceride levels must be checked periodically if propofol is administered for >24-48 hours. Neuromuscular blocking agents are rarely used because they may cause long-term weakness and increase length of ventilation although they may be indicated in some cases, such as with excessive shivering or cardiac arrest. Many patients are able to tolerate mechanical ventilation without sedation, and sedation should always be decreased to the minimal amount necessary as excess sedation may delay extubation.

Professional Role

Advanced practice registered nursing

Advanced practice registered nursing (APRN) – According to the NCSBN, the APRN is acting as a nurse with a foundation on information and proficiency that was obtained in basic nursing school. This nurse has a license to be an RN and has completed and received a diploma from graduate school in an APRN program that has been accredited from a nationwide accrediting body. This nurse has up-to-date certification from a nationwide certification board to work in the proper APRN area. Being an APRN defines the nurse as someone that has more responsibility, which may or may not come with more pay or gain for the nurse.

Some responsibilities include:
- Give professional education and leadership.
- Handle patient and medical center leadership.
- Support the patient and local area by keeping the ideal concerns for the patient or community.
- Assess reactions of involvement and how well medical routines are working.
- Be in touch with and act together with patients, patient relatives, and colleagues.
- Employ research; get and use new information and equipment.
- Educate others regarding APRN.

Advanced practice registered nurse (APRN) – Includes nurse anesthetists, nurse midwives, nurse practitioners, and clinical nurse specialists. These must have proper credentials and take the role of the main leadership in taking responsibility for the patient's care. Some other nurses who hold leadership responsibilities are not included under the term APRN. These nurses who are not included may have professional responsibilities but not in a clinical setting, such as teachers, administrators, or researchers, even though these nurses may have the same knowledge as an APRN. Someone that is not working in a client or family medical clinic cannot be an APRN. More than the 2–4 years of study that is needed to become a basic nurse is required to be an APRN. The APRN will have further study to meet the extra standards.

Advanced practice registered nurse (APRN) – This nurse leads the medical management of patients, supports the patient, is responsible for the patient goals and expense of care, medically handles patient conditions, dispenses information, leads, studies, gives advice, handles cases, and is a facilitator of modification.

Standards of practice – These are defined by the ANA (from 1998) and meant to be professional guidelines regarding the excellence of performance, service, and learning. They give the least amount of satisfactory work. It gives clients a way to determine the quality of the treatment that was given to them. There are broad and particular standards to the area of expertise. Some particular areas of expertise have their own standards as well, such as National Association of Pediatric Nursing Practitioners (NAPNP) and Association for Women's Health, Obstetric, and Neonatal Nurses (AWHONN). PNP has separate standards. All standards may be used in legal proceedings, but they are not originally meant for this purpose.

Certification for APRN:
- The government has no responsibility for certification. An agency or group verifies that the nurse has a license and has finished specific, set-forth standards as must be met in the particular area of expertise. It might be necessary to receive a state license or reimbursement. It is necessary to become an APRN in certain states.

Prescriptions:
- NPs and Certified Nurse-Midwives (CNM) have had the ability to write certain prescriptions since the mid-1970s. Since 1998, every state allows a degree of ability to write prescriptions. It is necessary that pharmacology instruction be included in the master's degree; the APRN has to get continued instruction to keep the authority to write prescriptions. Certain guidelines differ between the states. The range of what prescriptions are allowed is different between the states. Total ability for prescriptions includes the capability to get a federal DEA registration number.

Advanced practice registered nurse (APRN) – Responsibilities include but are not limited to the following:
- Evaluate the patient, produce and assess information; comprehend higher nursing practice in action at this rank.
- Assess many kinds of information; find differential diagnosis; determine proper medical care.
- Without supervision, determine how to handle difficult patient issues.
- Create a way to identify the condition, create objectives for the patient's medical management, and stipulate the medical routine or plan.
- Identify, set the routine for medical management, oversee, and give out the medical plan. This includes medicine and drugs as appropriate that fall inside of the APRN's area.
- Handle the patient's bodily and mental condition.
- Make sure there is protected and pertinent nursing being done, whether direct or indirect with regard to the patient.
- Keep protected and beneficial surroundings.

Credentials for APRN:
- Make sure there is answerability and conscientiousness for proficient work.
- Authenticates that the practitioner has received the correct instruction, has a license, and is certified.
- Compulsory to make sure that the local and national laws are followed. Recognizes the furthered scope for the APRN.
- Allows for needed ways for patients to make a grievance.
- Allows for responsibility for the community by making sure standards of practice are met.
- Debates between the State boards of Nursing and different education accrediting organizations were more heated in the 1990s due to more NP programs coming available.
- National task force with regard to the excellence of NP schools met in 1995. Many organizations were present.
- The government does not have a hand in credentialing.
- Credentials may be obtained through an AACN-acknowledged certifying body.

Mission and the vision of the AACN

The mission of the AACN is as follows:
- The American Association of Critical-Care Nurses (AACN) provides and inspires leadership to establish work and care environments that are respectful, healing, and humane. The AACN's key to success is through its members. Therefore, the AACN is committed to providing the highest quality resources to maximize nurses' contribution to caring for critically ill patients and their families.

The vision of the AACN is as follows:
- The AACN is dedicated to creating a health care system driven by the needs of patients and families where critical care professionals make their optimal contribution.

Standards of care for the Acute Care Nurse Practitioner (ACNP)

The ANA and the AACN have collaborated to provide published standards of care for the ACNP.
- Standard I states that the ACNP is responsible for collecting patient data.
- Standard II states that the ACNP is responsible for determining diagnoses by analyzing said data.
- Standard III states that the ACNP is responsible for identifying expected outcomes specific to the patient.
- Standard IV states that the ACNP is responsible for developing a care plan with specific interventions.
- Standard V states that the ACNP is responsible for implementing patient interventions.
- Standard VI states that the ACNP is responsible for evaluating the progress of the patient.

Standards of professional performance

The ANA and the AACN collaborated to publish a set of standards of professional performance for the ANCP as follows:
- Standard I states that the ACNP will systematically evaluate the quality and effectiveness of acute care nursing as a practice.
- Standard II states that the ACNP will use available organizational resources (e.g., publications, conferences) to aid in patient care.
- Standard III states that the ACNP will use professional practice standards to evaluate his or her own practice.
- Standard IV states that the ACNP will maintain current acute care knowledge.
- Standard V states that the ACNP will contribute to the professional development of colleagues.
- Standard VI states that the ACNP will make ethical decisions and act accordingly.
- Standard VII states that the ACNP will form collaborations in providing patient care.
- Standard VIII states that the ACNP will use research findings in his or her practice.
- Standard IX states that the ACNP will deliver patient care safely and effectively.

Values set forth by the AACN

In addition to its mission and vision, the AACN has also published a set of values intended for all AACN members to uphold. These values state that the AACN member will:

1. Be accountable for basing his or her practice on ethical actions and principles.
2. Advocate changes in the AACN organization that benefit patients and their families.
3. Practice with integrity, including honest communication, loyalty, and the honoring of promises and commitments.
4. Communicate and cultivate relationships with other AACN members.
5. Assume a leadership role, promoting strategic thinking, planning, and problem solving.
6. Meet and/or exceed all standards and expectations.
7. Remain a fair, impartial, and responsible leader.
8. Continue to make contributions through learning, questioning, and critical thinking.
9. Promote innovative thinking.
10. Remain committed and passionate about the organization, and inspire others to do the same.

Scope of Practice

The ACNP's Scope of Practice identifies a number of areas in which the ACNP should be competent. The ACNP is expected to have an extensive working knowledge base, and he or she is also expected to have excellent communication skills. The ability to perform both a patient health history and a physical examination are central to the ACNP's scope of practice, as is the ability to both order and interpret laboratory tests and diagnostic procedures. In addition, the ACNP is expected to be able to perform certain invasive procedures, such as intensive wound care, to remove drains and staples, and to assist in surgical procedures. The ACNP is required to prescribe drugs, and monitor the effects of those drugs during the course of treatment. The ACNP must be organized, enthusiastic, intuitive, inventive, and respectful towards patients, families, and other health care professionals.

The ACNP's scope of practice is dependent on each state and what the APRN in this position can do beneath the Nurse Practice Act for that state. The scope gives guidelines instead of particular directives. There is a big range, depending on the state. Many times the scope is founded on what is allowed legally both in the state and in the nation. The initial Scope of Practice for PNPs occurred in 1983 by the National Association of Pediatric Nurse Practitioners. This has been updated in 1990 and in 2000. Scope is always changing and improving.

Nursing practice acts – See the NCSBN Web site to find the complete list of state practice acts (not for every state, but 31 states are included): http://www.ncsbn.org. An authorizing board of nursing is available in every state to lead statutes with regard to licenses for an RN. They have responsibility for how titles are used, scope of work, and how to handle discipline cases. Nurse practice acts come out of statutory law.

Nurse Practitioner Guidelines

Curriculum guidelines for becoming a nurse practitioners are updated from time to time. The National Association of Nurse Practitioner Faculties (NONPF) put out a written curriculum plan for nurse practitioners in 1990, and was most recently updated in 2006. The basic graduate nurse has to complete the basic courses. An advanced practice RN has to complete the basic advanced courses. Each APRN will take classes that are distinctive to the kind of APRN that will be his/her specialty in order to better serve the patients. Theoretical study for the APRN includes Benner's model of expert practice from 1985, Calkin's model of advanced nursing practice from 1984, and Shuler's model of NP practice.

Nurse practitioner's policy expertise – The most important is for the nurse practitioner to get political allies. Having political friends that can make decisions (i.e., in the legislature) lets the nurse practitioner contribute and stay up to date about issues.

Three main areas that are vital for increasing what the nurse practitioner can do – Write prescriptions, reimbursement rights, and range of practice that is allowed under the law.

ICD-9-CM – International Classification of Diseases, 9th Edition; this has diagnostic codes that tell what medical problem, sickness, or harm the medical attention is for; utilized with billing insurance companies.

CPT – Current Procedural Terminology; these codes tell what procedure or medical attention was done; there are more than 7000. Both Medicare and state Medicaid carriers have to utilize these codes under the law.

HCPC – Health Care Financing Administration Common Procedure Coding System; this is utilized to make an account of supplies and medical tools.

Clinical practice guiding principles and practice

Clinical practice guiding principles and practice are needed so that the NP and the patient will know what is suitable with regard to medical treatment. It is different from state to state because of the different nurse practice acts for the states. Publications and notable references may be used to determine protocol needs. For instance, in pediatric care, with regard to guidelines for prevention of medical conditions, guidelines include Bright Futures (MCHB), Guidelines for Adolescent Preventative Services (AMA) and Guide to Preventative Services. As examples for pediatric care guidelines for sicknesses, there are asthma (NIH, AAP), hearing screening (NIH, AAP), HIV (AHRQ), otitis media including effusion (AHRQ), pain (AHRQ), and sickle cell disease (AHRQ).

Medicaid

Medicaid – 1965 Title XIX Social Security Act allowed for Medicaid. It is a federal/state matching plan, and federal is in charge of supervision. The money for it comes from federal and state taxes, and 50%–83% is funded by federal. Each state is able to put more services on the list and they may put restrictions (to a point) on federally directed aid. Patients who get Medicaid cannot get a bill for the aid, but states are able to give them small co-payments or deductibles for particular types of help.

Although Medicaid does not provide for everyone that lives under the federal poverty rate, some patients have to be covered under the federal government rules. These patients include:

- Patients who have gotten Aid to Families with Dependent Children (AFDC) (each state makes its own criterion for this).
- Patients that are older than 65, sightless, or have complete disability can get monetary help because of the Federal Supplemental Security income (SSI).
- Pregnant women are covered for pregnancy –associated help; children younger than 6 years of age who live in families that are up to 133% of the federal poverty level.
- Kids born following September of 1983 that live in families at or under the federal poverty level.

Medicare

Medicare – Federally directed; begun in 1965; gives health insurance to elderly patients and to patients with disabilities. The patient who is covered will get hospital, doctor, and further medical attention as needed. The amount that a patient makes is not a factor for eligibility. The two types are Medicare Part A and Medicare Part B – Supplementary Medical Insurance (SMI).

Medicare Part A – Anyone 65 years of age or older that is eligible to get Social Security is automatically enrolled even if still working. Patients are able to get Social Security if they or their spouse put money into the system by way of working for at least 40 quarters. If the patient has less than 40 quarters of work, Medicare Part A requires a payment each month. If the patient is not yet 65 but has a complete disability which will be there for the rest of their life, Medicare Part A can be used after receiving Social Security benefits for 2 years. A patient with ongoing renal disease who needs either dialysis or transplant can become eligible for Part A without waiting for 2 years.

Medicare Part A – Includes partial expenses for hospitalization, partial skilled nursing home expenses, and does not include custodial care. For home health, all of skilled care is covered, 80% of approved expenses for medical paraphernalia are covered, and hospice is generally totally covered. Hospitalization costs are determined by the anticipated expense of treatment for someone who has that particular issue. Every Medicare-covered patient who goes into the hospital becomes categorized by the diagnosis-related group (DRG). After that, the hospital gets payment for a preset sum for everyone who comes in with that particular DRG. When the expenses go beyond that, the hospital has to cover the extra expense. If the expenses are below that, the hospital gets to retain a certain percent of the extra money. An APRN will not be given money directly for working inside of a hospital.

Medicare Part B – The patient has to pay by the month. There are some who have a low enough salary that are entitled to have this month-to-month payment be paid by Medicaid. This program is paid for by general federal revenue and by these month-to-month payments. The program covers 80% of the authorized expense for any medical attention that is required (following a yearly deductible). This includes doctor visits, physical therapy, occupational therapy, speech therapy, medical paraphernalia, assessments, and certain types of prevention treatments like Pap smears, mammograms, and hepatitis B, pneumococcal, and influenza vaccinations.

APRN Medicare reimbursement – Legislation is from 1997; APRNs get 85% of doctor fee schedules if they are sending invoices by themselves with an APRN billing number. A doctor's management is not needed. If the APRN is under a doctor's management, the doctor's practice can get the total amount of the regular doctor's invoice. This is under the

"Incident to" rules. And APRN has to have a current RN license for the state in which he/she practices, and the APRN has to meet the criteria to do NP work for primary medical attention NP. There has to be a degree from a official educational facility in the proper area, and there has to include a minimum of one academic year which involves a minimum of 4 months of education in classes and a final outcome of a degree, diploma or certificate OR the person has to have productively finished an official advanced practice instructional curriculum and have worked doing this extended position for a minimum of a year inside the year and a half prior to February 8, 1978.

Medicare for the APRN's services in a skilled nursing facility – If the APRN does work in a skilled nursing facility (SNF) or a nursing home that is in an urban region (urban regions are legally distinct), then Medicare money may be acquired. Medicare will pay reimbursements for an APRN's work done in SNF if it is not a defined rural region with a justifiable amount of payment. That expanse cannot be more than what a doctor's fee would be for work. The money is paid to the APRN's manager.

Malpractice reimbursement – An APRN has to be reimbursed. It does not make a difference if the APRN works alone, has a joint practice together, works in a hospital, or works in managed care. Many times federal policies for Medicaid or Medicare are used to find out what the pay will be for private-pay insurance. Although the federal government includes directives that promote paying the medical worker (who is not a doctor) in a noncircuitous manner, it is common to find that there are obstacles due to state rules and regulations.

Centers for Medicare and Medicaid Services (CMS):
- Used to be called Health Care Financing and Administration (HCFA).
- Administration for many federal plans such as Medicare, Medicaid, HIPAA, CLIA, and State children's health insurance program (SCHIP).
- See http://cms.hhs.gov for more information.

Advanced practice nurses – May be paid in one of these ways:
- Fee-for-service.
- Episodic.
- Capitation, PPO, HMO.

Medicaid and Medicare Omnibus Budget Reconciliation Act

Medicaid and Medicare for APRNs – In 1989, the Omnibus Budget Reconciliation Act (OBRA) made it obligatory for there to be Medicaid reimbursement payment to certified children and family nurse practitioners. This started on the first day of July 1990. The practitioner has to only do what is inside of the range of what is allowed in that state. The practitioner does not have to be responsible for the management of or be linked to a doctor or another medical professional. The amount to be paid is contingent upon the state, but is in the scope of 70%– 100% of the fee-for-service doctor Medicaid amount. Children and family nurse practitioners are allowed to send an invoice to Medicaid in a noncircuitous manner following getting a provider number from the Medicaid agency for the particular state. Each state can choose to make laws letting them make Medicaid reimbursements go to more categories of NP that are not found in the federal mandates.

Incident to

"Incident to" – With regard to the work done which is essential but incidental as a portion of a doctor's personal and expert work during identification of a condition or while giving medical attention for harm or a condition. The work has to happen when the patient is in the managed care of a doctor. The APRN has to be working for that doctor's group. The work has to happen while the patient is receiving medical attention from a doctor and follow-up work has to be in such a way that the doctor is a current contributor and is supervising the medical attention. Active personal management does not indicate that this doctor has to stay in the identical room with the APRN, but the doctor does have to be somewhere in that office area and accessible to help and manage during the APRN's medical attention.

Third party compensation

Covered for NP services – Restricted to work that an NP is allowed to do in that state, work that the NP normally does, and work that the NP has been trained, given instruction on, and fulfilled any conditions for as determined by the Secretary of Health and Human Services. This work is covered with Part B if/when an MD or Doctor of Osteopathy did the same work it would have been under a doctor's services, when the NP is allowed under the law to do the work in that state, if the work is done in collaboration with an MD or DO, and the work would otherwise be disqualified for coverage due to a legal exclusion.

Third parties:
- Private insurance – Will reimburse according to contract; particular for each state insurance commission.
- Civilian Health and Medical Program of the United States (CHAMPUS).
- Federal medical plan – Used by patients in the armed forces, their dependents that may be living beyond a time when they have died, their families, or retirees.
- Federal Employees Health Benefit Program (FEHBP).

Malpractice insurance

Malpractice insurance – This will not shield an APRN from being liable for giving medical attention with no license to do so in a case where the APRN is acting beyond what he or she is legally allowed to do in the particular state. The National Practitioner Data Bank gathers data regarding actions in opposition to medical professionals. Nurses are included in the data bank. Malpractice insurance may be occurrence coverage or claims-made coverage. Occurrence coverage is for an instance that happened when the policy was in effect, even if the date of discovery or the claim was filed after a point when the coverage ended. Claims-made coverage is for claims made inside the time that the policy was in effect, even if the instance happened at another time. Optional tail coverage contract makes the coverage go even further on a claims-made policy so that any subsequent claims that may come up as time goes by are covered even if the basic claims-made coverage time is over.

Coordination of care

Good coordination of care results in safe and effective health care for the patient. By establishing an effective care coordination plan, the health care team will also make sure that each individual team member's job is easier; this contributes to greater job satisfaction, more time for patient interaction, and less room for error, which all together result in better patient care. Coordination of care is an especially important part of the role of the APRN, because APRNs are often the first health care workers that the patient has any contact with, and they are also the health care workers that the patient has the most contact with, which means that they are in the best position for establishing care coordination.

Coordination of care is an important part of ensuring that the patient receives the best treatment possible. APRNs are a vital part of the coordination of care. APRN care coordination is defined as actions that are initiated by the APRN and involve patients, their family members, and other members of the health care team. These actions are meant to manage and correct the way that care is administered to the patient, such as changing the sequence of actions (making sure that the patient is on the ward when the phlebotomist comes to draw labs, instead of sending the patient to CT and having the phlebotomist come back, for example) to optimize the effectiveness of patient care from the time the patient is admitted to the hospital until the time the patient is discharged.

Interdisciplinary team

The formation of an interdisciplinary team is an important part of the coordination of care. An interdisciplinary team consists of health care workers (physicians, APRNs, social workers, and others) who specialize in different areas of medicine, and may work in different areas of the hospital; the team is formed because these health care workers, though in different specialties, share a common patient population and common patient care goals. Through the formation of the interdisciplinary team, active communication is established between the members of the team, their patients, and the patients' families. An interdisciplinary team may include, for example, a cardiologist, a cardiovascular surgeon, a coronary care unit APRN, and an ultrasound technician.

In addition to the interdisciplinary team approach, there are several other recognized approaches to patient care. One of these approaches is the independent medical management approach, in which one clinician works alone (for the most part) with limited contact with and clinical input from other clinicians. Another approach is the multidisciplinary care approach, in which each health care worker involved in the patient care works independently of the others involved in the care of the patient; these health care workers do not collaborate, but rather each is assigned a specific task to perform. The third approach is consultative; in this case, the clinician assumes the majority of patient care, but may request consultations from other clinicians.

The cognitive model of APRN care coordination is a guide to help APRNs form an effective plan for the coordination of patient care. APRN-patient communication, patient monitoring, task monitoring, and communication within the interdisciplinary care team are all important factors for the APRN to consider when assessing the overall situation; the APRN can gain a greater sense of awareness about the situation by examining all of these factors. Once the situation has been assessed, the APRN can develop a plan of action for him or herself and the other members of the interdisciplinary team, and the team can begin carrying out the necessary tasks. External factors that affect the development and execution of the care plan include the individual workload and the complexity of the tasks.

The interdisciplinary team approach to care coordination is beneficial to the patient in several ways. First, the quality of patient care is improved because several different medical services are involved in the care of the patient, and each service is familiar with the patient's situation as a result of increased communication with other health care workers. The interdisciplinary team approach also allows the patient to have a more active role in his or her care because of the emphasis on communication between the patient and all the team members. When the clinicians work together, they also make better use of time spent with the patient, so that the patient is not subjected to lengthy history-taking sessions and redundant testing by unaware clinicians.

Acting as an APRN preceptor for students is yet another role that the APRN is expected to perform, and this can be a difficult task for an APRN who is already strapped for time. When the APRN is a member of an interdisciplinary team, he or she will have more time to spend teaching students; at the same time, the student will find it easier to learn from a coordinated care system, rather than one that is hectic and confusing. The student (and the APRN) will both benefit from being exposed to health care workers who specialize in other areas. The communicative environment of the interdisciplinary team will also encourage student participation.

In addition to being beneficial to the patient, the interdisciplinary team approach is also very beneficial to the APRN or health care professional. Perhaps the most significant benefit of this approach to care coordination is that it shifts the focus from acute patient care to long-term care that is prevention-centric. This has the added benefit of increasing professional satisfaction for the APRN, because he or she will feel that a difference is being made, and the reduction in stress makes the work environment more comfortable. Another benefit for the APRN is that when he or she is working in coordination with other specialties, he or she has more time to focus on his or her own specialty area without having to do extraneous, redundant work. The reduction in time spent performing unnecessary tasks means that the APRN has more time to learn new skills.

Analytical decision making

An analytical decision is one that is made after a systematic review and analysis of all factors involved in the decision; concentration and awareness are important in the analytical decision-making process. In contrast with an intuitive decision, the analytical decision takes longer to make, because it is not automatic. The analysis is based on an in-depth look at all factors, and is based on scientific evidence (in other words, it is based on the outcomes of previous similar situations). Because an analytical decision is based on scientific evidence and facts, the outcome of the decision has a high predictive value; this means that by looking at previous outcomes, it is possible to predict the current outcome. Because the clinician has so carefully reviewed all factors, he or she will most likely not experience the emotional anxiety associated with an intuitive decision.

Intuitive decision-making

When a clinician makes an intuitive decision, he or she is making a decision not necessarily based on fact, but more so because it feels like the right decision. Of course, in most cases, one would not want a doctor making decisions this way, although in certain cases (say, a choice between 2 different types of treatment, each of which has the same general risks, or when all other options have been exhausted), it may be necessary. Although these decisions are not based on an analysis of the facts, there is something to be said about the so-called "gut instinct," which years of training and experience can hone. These decisions are made without spending a lot of time on the process of decision making; though they are based on experience, the clinician may suffer some degree of anxiety about the decision and its outcome.

Clinical decision-making

Although one would like to think that there isn't much variation in the clinical decision-making process, this simply is not true. The process, of course, will differ depending on the patient, the differential diagnosis, and the clinician. First, let's start with the clinician. The way that the clinician conducts the clinical decision-making process is influenced by the knowledge base of the clinician, as well as the level of his experience, the ability he possesses to think both critically and creatively, and the confidence that he has in his ability to make educated decisions. The acuity level of the patient is also a factor in the clinical decision-making process, as is the length of the differential. A time stressor is placed on the clinician when the condition of the patient is critical, and when there are more diseases that must be eliminated from the differential. An element of stress may also exist if the clinician has a high number of patients, especially if he has multiple high-acuity patients.

Aside from time (or lack thereof), there are other external or environmental stressors that may have an effect on the clinical decision-making process. One of these stressors is inadequate staffing. If the department does not have enough staff to handle the workload, or if there are not enough experienced staff members to help the less-experienced staff members, this can cause problems with the decision-making process, both by adding a time stressor, and by not providing enough resources for the staff. Another stressor that has an effect on the clinical decision-making process is the presence of strained interpersonal relationships; strained relationships may occur between 2 or more APRNs, between physicians, or between APRNs and physicians. Whatever the combination, a strained relationship between individuals who should be working together can negatively impact decision making.

Knowledge base, attention, and barriers to care

Knowledge base refers to the amount of working knowledge that is available to the practicing APRN; a new graduate, for example, will not have as broad a knowledge base as a veteran APRN. A new APRN may not be able to make confident clinical decisions, which can put the patient at risk; for this reason, it is important that there be more experienced APRNs available for consultation. Attention simply refers to the amount of attention that the APRN is dedicating to the patient and his or her complaints. Attention may be compromised by any number of things; for example, maybe the APRN is preoccupied by something outside of work. This can be detrimental to the patient as well; the APRN should always devote his or her full attention to the patient. There are many barriers that may compromise the safety of the patient as well. Perhaps there are not enough beds to keep up with new admissions, or maybe no one is available for an urgent consult.

Factors related to safety that may influence decision-making abilities

In 2005, Ebright et al published a study of factors related to safety and the decision-making ability of the APRN. Every clinical decision made by the APRN has an effect on the safety of the patient, and therefore any factor that influences the APRN's decision-making ability may adversely affect the patient. Ebright at al identified the following factors that influence decision-making and patient safety: knowledge base, attention, barriers to care, number of tasks, missing essential information, and behaviors that are not encouraging of productive thought. The presence of, or a change in, any of these factors can result in unnecessary harm for the patient.

Hollnagel's contextual control model

Hollnagel's contextual control model is a method that was devised in order to assess how team behavior is affected by the level of organization and by environmental factors. Hollnagel proposed that when working together, a team has 4 specific modes of action; these 4 modes are strategic, tactical, opportunistic, and scrambled. The contextual control model states that the mode of action of a team is affected by the level of planning, as well as the nature of the surrounding environment. If the team has a high level of planning, the associated mode of action is strategic; conversely, if the mode of action is scrambled, the team will likely be reactive to and distracted by the environment, rather than operating by a set plan.

Basic modes that the APRN may find him or herself in when coordinating patient care

There are three basic modes that the APRN may find him or herself in when coordinating patient care; these modes are based on the overall stress level at the time of planning. The first level is called steady-state mode; this is the mode that the APRN is in when the stress level is low to normal. The APRN does not feel overwhelmed and is able to handle tasks efficiently and effectively. The next level is called problem mode; in problem mode, the stress level is higher than the APRN may be able to handle by him or herself, and as such, he or she may find it necessary to delegate tasks to other members of the health care team. The third level, crisis mode, is a high-stress environment or situation where multiple people may be enlisted to help, as quick action is required.

Clinical challenging

"Clinical challenging" is defined as the questioning of a clinician by a APRN regarding another clinician's reasoning for making certain clinical decisions. The APRN has the opportunity to challenge the clinician on his or her decisions during patient rounds, when the clinician's explanation of his or her reasoning can benefit all of the members of the health care team who are present. The purpose of clinical challenging is for the clinician to employ critical thinking and critical decision making, rather than making decisions solely based on traditional treatment approaches. The critical thinking atmosphere promotes discussions about ongoing research that may be beneficial to the patient. If the clinician cannot provide an answer, he or she may search for information from recently published studies. APRNs may be hesitant to challenge other clinicians on their decisions, but it is an important part of the learning process, and it is important for the promotion of research and the improvement of patient care.

Quality improvement

Quality improvement (QI) – Accomplished through peer review or another form of assessment. In peer review, the approach is to acknowledge and prize the work nurses do. This shows the way toward better standards of work and puts off work that is not within what the practitioner can legally do. It heightens the quality of medical attention and gives a means for attaining answerability and conscientiousness. Another form of assessment may include an audit, question/answer or appraisal, or patient contentment question/answer or appraisal.

Risk management – Organizations and actions meant to acknowledge and intercede resulting in less chance of harm to a patient and ensuing claims in opposition to the medical attention workers. This is founded on the supposition that a lot of harm done to patients could be stopped from happening in the first place. Risk management is an assessment of places when legal responsibility is an issue, like patients, methods, or how accounts are maintained. Risk management also involves instruction used to lessen the chance of a problem in a recognized part.

Diagnostic-related groups

Diagnostic-related groups (DRGs) were instituted in 1982 as a way to classify patients who shared similar diseases and treatments for billing purposes, under the assumption that patients who shared symptoms and/or diseases use the same amount of resources and should be billed the same amount. There are approximately 500 different DRGs, and patients are placed into specific DRGs using International Classification of Disease (ICD) codes, along with specific patient information such as sex, age, and the presence of comorbidities. By placing patients into DRGs, Medicare is able to determine how much the hospital should be reimbursed for patient care. The institution of DRGs has changed the health care system from one that was provider-driven (meaning the individual clinician determined the billable amount) into one that is payer-driven (meaning that Medicare determines reimbursement).

APRN's role as an educator

The APRN's role as an educator spans 2 major groups: patients and their families, and colleagues. The APRN is required to educate patients about their illnesses and diseases; because patients may not possess much medical knowledge, it is important that the clinician provide information that is easily understandable. A properly educated patient is much better equipped to take care of him or herself, and can recognize potential health problems; the same applies to family members on whom the patient may rely for care. The APRN can provide this education through a meeting with the patient and his or her family, in which treatment options and other information are discussed. Supplemental books, pamphlets, and videos are also helpful. Concerning colleague education, the APRN may present information at rounds and conferences; he or she may also assume the role of preceptor for nursing students.

Goals of educating patients

The Joint Commission (1994) states that "the goal of educating the patient and family is to improve patient health outcomes by promoting recovery, speeding return to function, promoting health behavior, and appropriately involving the patient in his or her own health care decisions."

The needs assessment is a tool used by clinicians to determine what behaviors and information the patient needs to be educated about. Once the clinician has determined what the patient's specific needs are, he or she can begin to teach the patient and the patient's family the necessary behavior modifications and information. For the APRN, it is important to weed out the nonessential information, because the acute care environment does not allow time for this, and the nonessential information will detract from the information that is important for the patient's recovery.

Patient needs assessment

When the APRN conducts a patient needs assessment, he or she should find out as much information as possible regarding what the patient needs to know, as well as the best way to educate the patient so that the teaching-learning process is a success. There are a number of questions that should be answered during the patient needs assessment:
1. What information does the patient already know?
2. Has the patient/family had any previous experience with this particular health issue?
3. Does the patient have any cultural beliefs that may impact his or her behavior modification?
4. What is the patient's preferred learning style?
5. Can the patient read?
6. What resources are available for use in the teaching-learning process?
7. What are the teaching and learning preferences of the APRN?
8. What method should be used to evaluate behavior modification?
9. What will motivate the patient to change his or her behavior?
10. Are there any barriers to educating this patient?

WRAT as an assessment of literacy

Before the APRN can begin teaching the patient, he or she must formulate a teaching strategy that is appropriate for the patient. The APRN cannot formulate a teaching strategy until he or she is familiar with the patient's literacy level. There are several available tests that the APRN can use to evaluate the patient's literacy level. Once of these tests is the Wide Range Achievement Test (WRAT), in which the patient is given a list of words to read aloud, until he or she has made 10 mistakes in pronunciation. The patient's reading grade level is then determined by the number of words he or she has pronounced correctly.

Motivating patients to learn behavior modification

It can be difficult for the APRN to motivate the patient to take an active role in his or her treatment and recovery; the patient is in the hospital, sick, and probably already overwhelmed. There are several ways in which the APRN can motivate the patient to learn without adding to the burden. The use of visual aids is a great way to motivate the patient and hold his or her attention and interest. Rewards and praise are also great motivators; if the patient does not have much of a support system at home, this is especially important. The patient will be more likely to learn when he or she wants to know something, so it is important for the APRN to respond to all of the patient's questions fully and in a timely manner. Teach the material to the patient beginning with easy material first, and then progressing to complex. This ensures that the patient can achieve his or her goals, which is a great motivator.

Evaluation

The evaluation process is important, and it is beneficial not only to the patient, but to the educator as well. Regarding the patient, evaluation helps the patient figure out how to correct his or her behavior, and it also reinforces correct behavior modifications. Regarding the educator, the evaluation process determines whether the education provided is accurate. There are 2 ways in which adult patients can be evaluated: direct evaluation and indirect evaluation. Direct evaluation occurs when the educator directly observes the patient engaging in the modified behavior. When direct evaluation is not possible, an indirect approach is taken; in this case, the patient can be evaluated through his or her answers to written and/or oral questions.

REALM and TOFLA tests

It is important, in addition to establishing a base literacy level, for the APRN to establish the patient's medical literacy level; this gives the APRN a better understanding of what the patient does know, and what the patient needs to know, about health care. The Rapid Estimate of Adult Literacy in Medicine (REALM) test is somewhat similar in style to the WRAT test; the patient is given a list of medical-related words and asked to read them. The patient's literacy score is based on the number of words he or she can pronounce. The Test for Functional Health Literacy in Adults (TOFLA) is a more comprehensive test; in addition to measuring medical literacy, it assesses the patient's medical reading comprehension and understanding of numerical values related to medicine.

Andragogy

Andragogy (which comes from the Greek for "man-leading") is defined as the process of engaging adults in the learning process.

A study conducted by Malcolm Knowles states that there are 2 basic conditions that are necessary for the education of adults. The first condition is that the educator must facilitate a climate of collaboration; in other words, the student-adult must not feel that the educator is "superior" and the student himself "inferior." There must be a mutual respect, and the student-adult must be able to trust the educator. The second condition is that the student-adult must have an active role in the learning process; he or she should be included in the needs assessment process, as well as in self-evaluation.

Basic learning theories

There are, traditionally, three basic learning theories: the behaviorist theory, the cognitive theory, and the social cognitive (or constructive) theory. The behaviorist theory is based on the assumption that learning is a modification of behavior based on conditioning (behavior reinforcement). Positive reinforcement is seen as a powerful moderator of learning and behavior modification. The cognitive theory is based on the idea that learning is motivated by the need for certain knowledge, and not through a change in behavior. Under the cognitive theory, an individual will be motivated to learn only the things that he or she feels are necessary to accomplish his or her life goals. The social cognitive theory is based on the idea that an individual will be more likely to modify his or her behavior if he or she has a role model to emulate.

Techniques to be used when teaching adults

Knowles includes several general techniques for teaching adults as part of his study of andragogy. These techniques directly correlate to Knowles' assumptions of adult teaching; once the assumptions are understood, the teaching-learning techniques should be obvious. The first general technique is for the educator to teach adult learners based on their own past experiences. The second technique is the use of problem-based or problem-oriented learning activities, such as case studies or role-playing situational activities. The third technique is for the educator to share the responsibility of teaching with the learners, giving each learner an active role in the educational process. Adult learners should also be given an active role in evaluations. The fourth technique, aimed at keeping the adult learner interested, is to employ a variety of learning techniques and teaching strategies.

Teaching a patient with disabilities

It is to be expected that the APRN will frequently encounter patients with disabilities. It is important that the APRN is able to recognize what modifications he or she needs to make to his or her teaching strategies when addressing a patient with a disability. King and Cheatham have established a set of general guidelines for the APRN to follow when interacting with a disabled patient. The first guideline is to maintain eye contact with the patient; it is important that the patient not feel uncomfortable, and it is important that the patient trust the caregiver. The next guideline is that, during the teaching process, the APRN should always address the patient, not the patient's family members. The APRN should also remember to encourage active participation from the patient, whether through spoken or written communication. The APRN should also ask the patient if he or she requires any assistance with anything before providing that assistance. Lastly, but equally important, maintain a normal tone of voice.

Videos

Videos are a useful adjunct to teaching as they reduce the time needed for one-on-one instruction (increasing cost-effectiveness). Passive presentation of videos, such as in the waiting area, has little value, but focused viewing in which the nurse discusses the purpose of the video presentation prior to viewing and then is available for discussion after viewing can be very effective. Patients and/or families are often nervous about learning patient care and are unsure of their abilities, so they may not focus completely when the nurse is presenting information. Allowing the patients/families to watch a video demonstration or explanation first and allowing them to stop or review the video presentation can help them to grasp the fundamentals before they have to apply them, relieving some of the anxiety them may be experiencing. Videos are much more effective than written materials for those with low literacy or poor English skills. The nurse should always be available to answer questions and discuss the material after the patients/families finish viewing.

Teaching patients with low literacy skills

When educating a patient with low literacy skills, the APRN must take special care to ensure that the material is presented in a way that the patient can easily understand. Because the patient may not understand them, it is not possible for the APRN to hand the patient a bunch of pamphlets about the disease and treatment. Instead, the APRN may have to devote more time to a discussion with the patient. The APRN should frequently ask the patient questions as a method of evaluation to make sure that the patient understands the information. Other educational materials, such as videos, audiotapes, and pictures, may also be used to supplement discussions with the patient.

Person-centered care

"Person-centered care" is a patient-care model that was developed by Allen Barbour; in his model, which is somewhat a critique of the standard medical model, he states that person-centered care "refer[s] specifically to becoming familiar with the patient's personal situation in its crucial relationship to the source of illness." The APRN's role in risk assessment as outlined by Neuman framework definitely allows room for the idea of person-centered care, because it includes a look not only at the patient's physiological stressors, but also at his or her psychologic, social, and cultural stressors. Often times these stressors are brushed aside to assess pathophysiological issues. The APRN is in a unique position in that he or she has more interaction with the patient on a personal level, and can help identify these other stressors that have just as significant an impact on the patient's illness progression and recovery.

Therapeutic communication

Communication is important in establishing a good nurse-patient relationship. Therapeutic communication is any exchange between a health care worker and a patient; however, the goal of therapeutic communication is to foster interactions with the patient in which the patient grows and moves towards his or her treatment goals. It is important that the APRN is understanding of the fears and feelings of the patient, and can ease the patient's worries through open communication. The APRN should be available for support, and should provide any information the patient needs. The APRN should also provide feedback along the way, creating an environment where the patient feels comfortable asking questions. The patient needs to know that the APRN is listening, and that his or her concerns and ideas are being heard. These elements help establish therapeutic communication between the APRN and the patient.

Active listening on the part of the APRN (and on the part of the patient, as well) is an important part of the therapeutic communication process. For the APRN, this is referred to as "patient-centered" listening. It is important that the APRN not just hear but understand what the patient is saying, and it is important that the patient knows that the APRN is listening. When interacting with the patient, the APRN should allow the patient to do more of the talking; this, in addition to maintaining eye contact and using affirmative nonverbal communication (e.g., nodding), shows the patient that he or she is respected. The APRN should remember to keep his or her focus on the patient. By showing the patient that he or she is respected and valued, the APRN establishes the groundwork for effective therapeutic communication.

When the APRN is interviewing the patient, there are a number of ways in which he or she can make the patient feel more comfortable, and assure the patient that he or she is being heard. Eye contact and affirmative, receptive nonverbal communication is important. Another important technique is restating; to use this technique, the APRN should restate part of the patient's last comment before asking the next question. For example, the patient has described to the APRN that he has been experiencing dull, constant headaches for the past week that become more painful at night. The APRN's next question may be "You say that the pain becomes more severe at night. Is it associated with any specific activity, such as lying down?" By restating some of the patient's previous statement, the APRN shows that he or she is listening to the patient, and taking his answers seriously.

Clarification

When being interviewed, the patient may not always be able to express him or herself clearly; maybe he or she is frightened, or embarrassed, or just overwhelmed at the situation, and this is to be expected. When the APRN senses that the patient is having a hard time explaining something, he or she may ask the patient for clarification. The best way to do this is to ask the patient more specific questions, so that more specific answers can be given. The patient may be vague in his or her answers, especially because he or she is not sure what information is important to the APRN, and what information is not. By asking specific questions, the APRN is better able to understand the patient, and the patient has a better idea what the APRN needs to know. The APRN should always ask questions if he or she does not understand something the patient has said.

Focusing

The APRN walks a fine line when attempting to establish a relationship with his or her patient; there must be mutual respect and understanding, and the patient must feel comfortable communicating with the APRN. The APRN must be able to gather important information from the patient without being brusque or demanding. Some patients may be nervous and talkative, and may want to talk about other topics in an effort to avoid discussing the issue or issues at hand. The APRN may find it necessary to focus the patient on specific areas of discussion; this should be done tactfully, so as not to make the patient feel that he or she is not important. Questions such as "do you mind if I ask you a few questions about how you are feeling about the current situation?" or "is there anything specific you would like to discuss regarding your illness?" are appropriate.

Reflection

Reflection is somewhat similar to restating, in that part of the purpose of the technique is to demonstrate to the patient that the nurse is listening to what he or she is saying. Reflection refers to an understanding of the patient's feelings, in addition to an understanding of what he or she is saying. When an APRN employs reflection as a communicative technique, he or she is paying attention not only to the patient's words, but also to the patient's actions and affect. The APRN can then ask the patient about his or her feelings regarding the discussion. This demonstrates to the patient that the APRN is understanding of and interested in the patient, and that the APRN is empathetic. It is important that the APRN and patient are comfortable enough with each other to reflect on feelings before the APRN attempts to use reflection as a technique so as not to make the patient uncomfortable.

Silence

Although therapeutic communication is focused on active interaction between the APRN and the patient, silence can be an important part of the therapeutic relationship. In some cases, silence can be beneficial to the relationship. For example, if the patient is extremely talkative, silence on the part of the APRN can indicate to the patient that the APRN is listening and taking him or her seriously. In this case, silence is welcomed by the patient. At certain times during communication, silence can be effective, especially if it is meant to provide the patient an opportunity to reflect. If the patient is quiet, depressed, or made uncomfortable by prolonged silence, then silence on the part of the APRN could be detrimental to the relationship.

Value clarification

A value is a belief possessed by an individual that has the power to motivate that individual's behavior. Values can be spiritual, cultural, or religious; an individual can formulate his or her own set of values based on education, and on his or her own life experiences. These values can then serve as a guideline for that individual's future decisions. Some values, however, may guide behaviors and decisions without the individual's awareness of their existence. The process of value clarification can help an individual uncover beliefs that may be negatively influencing behavior; once these beliefs and values have been uncovered, the individual can analyze and reevaluate them.

Theme identification

As the APRN has more opportunities to communicate with the patient, he or she may notice that the patient seems to be more interested in talking about some things than others, or more concerned with certain things than others. Active listening and engagement help the APRN to be more perceptive and identify specific things that are important to the patient. This process is called "theme identification"; by identifying these areas of importance, the APRN can better understand the patient's concerns. Asking the patient about these concerns ("You have mentioned being interested in alternatives to surgery, are you worried about having to undergo surgery?") shows the patient that he or she is being taken seriously, and gives him or her the opportunity to discuss specific fears and concerns more freely.

Informing and suggesting

Informing is a communicative technique whereby the APRN shares facts and information with the patient; it is important that the APRN conveys this information in such a way that the patient does not feel that he or she is being given advice by the APRN. An APRN informing a patient about something is considered to be part of the process of patient education, and the patient should be aware that the APRN is providing him or her with facts, not opinions. Suggesting, on the other hand, is more of an advice-giving technique; the APRN may provide the patient with alternative options, in addition to offering his or her opinion about which options are best for the patient.

Transference

Transference is a situation in which the patient projects feelings and attitudes towards the APRN that he or she has towards another individual (usually an authority figure) in his or her life. For example, if the APRN reminds a patient of his mother, with whom he has a poor relationship, he may treat the APRN as he would treat his mother. This is an unconscious reaction on the part of the patient, and can severely impede the therapeutic communication between the APRN and the patient. If the APRN suspects that he or she is being transferred upon by the patient, he or she must resolve the situation before the therapeutic relationship can resume.

Supporting families of dying patients

Families of dying patients often do not receive adequate support from nursing staff that feel unprepared for dealing with families' grief and unsure of how to provide comfort, but families may be in desperate need of this support:

Before death
- Stay with the family and sit quietly, allowing them to talk, cry, or interact if they desire.
- Avoid platitudes, "His suffering will be over soon."
- Avoid judgmental reactions to what family members say or do and realize that anger, fear, guilt, and irrational behavior are normal responses to acute grief and stress.
- Show caring by touching the patient and encouraging family to do the same.
- Note: Touching hands, arms, or shoulders of family members can provide comfort, but follow clues of the family.
- Provide referrals to support groups if available.

Time of death
- Reassure family that all measures have been taken to ensure the patient's comfort.
- Express personal feeling of loss, "She was such a sweet woman, and I'll miss her" and allow family to express feelings and memories. Provide information about what is happening during the dying process, explaining death rales, Cheyne-Stokes respirations, etc.
- Alert family members to imminent death if they are not present. Assist to contact clergy/spiritual advisors.
- Respect feelings and needs of parents, siblings, and other family.

After death
- Encourage parents/family members to stay with the patient as long as they wish to say goodbye.
- Use the patient's name when talking to the family.
- Assist family to make arrangements, such as contacting funeral home.
- If an autopsy is required, discuss with the family and explain when it will take place.
- If organ donation is to occur, assist the family to make arrangements. Encourage family members to grieve and express emotions. Send card or condolence note.

Patient advocacy

Patient advocacy is often seen as a moral obligation that the APRN must fulfill, and is a rewarding part of the APRN's job; however, patient advocacy can be difficult in certain situations. One barrier to advocacy is a feeling of powerlessness on the part of the APRN; sometimes it may feel as if it is the APRN against the world, especially if the APRN has no support; lack of support in general is another barrier. A lack of knowledge of the law is another barrier; certain laws may exist, though the APRN may not be aware of them. If the APRN and his or her peers are lacking in time, communication, or motivation, advocacy will also prove difficult. Another problem that APRNs frequently encounter is the risk associated with advocacy; included are disagreeing with other APRNs and physicians, and lack of legal support for the advocate.

Resistance

Resistance from the patient is a serious roadblock in the APRN-patient relationship, and stalls therapeutic communication. There are several reasons why a patient may become resistant to communication with the APRN:
1. The patient feels that the APRN became familiar too quickly, or probed too deeply into the patient's feelings too quickly.
2. The APRN has not presented him or herself as a good role model for the patient.
3. The patient feels that there is a lack of respect from the APRN.
4. The patient does not feel comfortable communicating with the APRN because of either intentional or unintentional nonverbal cues from the APRN (no eye contact, for example).
5. The patient feels that he or she may gain something by not engaging in a therapeutic relationship with the APRN; this is sometimes called secondary gain, an example being that a patient wishes to remain in the hospital because he is homeless, and he does not want to improve himself and be discharged.

Hostile transference and dependent reaction transference

Transference typically manifests in one of two ways: hostile transference or dependent reaction transference. Hostile transference may be expressed by the patient in various ways. If the patient is outwardly hostile, he or she may be uncooperative and negative; he or she may also be critical of the APRN, and challenge the APRN's decisions, or he or she may just ignore the APRN completely. If the patient internalizes his or her hostility, the APRN may see this as depression. Dependent reaction transference is much different in that the patient sees the APRN as all-knowing and all-important, and assumes a pattern of submission and dependence; in these cases, the patient depends on the APRN for everything, and the APRN may quickly become overwhelmed with demands.

Patient relationship boundary violations

There are various ways in which the APRN-patient relationship can be violated; most of them are obvious, but some of them may not be, especially if the APRN is naïve. It is important that the APRN not violate any boundaries of his or her relationship with the patient, and therefore the APRN should familiarize him or herself with the types of boundaries that exist in the APRN-patient relationship:
1. Role boundaries: The APRN should perform his or her duties as an APRN, and nothing else.
2. Time boundaries: The APRN should not visit the patient at 3 AM if there is no therapeutic reason.
3. Place and space boundaries
4. Money boundaries
5. Gift and service boundaries: The APRN should not accept any gifts from the patient.
6. Clothing boundaries: The APRN should dress professionally and appropriately.
7. Language boundaries: The APRN should not use offensive language.
8. Self-disclosure boundaries
9. Post-discharge social boundaries
10. Physical contact boundaries

Access to care

Access to care is often difficult for patients in nonemergent clinical situations. The patient may go to the emergency department and find him or herself waiting for hours and hours while people with more emergent problems are triaged ahead of them, leaving the patient both sick and frustrated. The patient may instead decide to call his or her primary care physician, only to find that he or she cannot be seen until after the weekend, leaving the patient to fend for himself. It is important for clinics, hospitals, and doctor's offices to provide patient-centered access to care. The characteristics of patient-centered care include availability of treatment for the patient, appropriateness of care, the ability of the patient to have a preference regarding care, and timeliness of care.

Counseling for children regarding injury prevention

Injury prevention counseling is a strong recommendation for the birth to 10-year age group, owing to the fact that motor vehicle accidents and other unintentional accidents are leading causes of death for this population. Children (and their parents) should be advised to use car safety seats until the age of 5 (this is subject to state law, however, as some states require the use of booster seats until a certain height or age is reached). After the age of 5, standard safety belts should always be used. When biking, skating, or skateboarding, a helmet should always be worn; these activities should not take place in the street. Parents should be advised to become CPR certified. They should also be advised to keep drugs, poisons, guns and other weapons, and matches out of the reach of children; to install smoke detectors and plan an escape route in the event of fire; and to make sure that stairs, windows, and pools are safe for children.

Counseling for individuals in the 11 to 24-year age population

Individuals in the 11 to 24-year age group should be provided counseling in the following areas: injury prevention, substance use, sexual behavior, diet and exercise, and dental health. Regarding injury prevention, these individuals should be advised about the use of seat belts and helmets. Counseling about the dangers of drug, alcohol, and tobacco use is also important. This age group should be educated regarding safe sex practices and sexually transmitted disease prevention, including abstinence, condoms, and other contraceptive devices. Education should also be provided concerning the importance of a balanced diet (avoiding too much fat and cholesterol, eating a variety of grains, fruits, and vegetables, limiting sugar intake) and regular exercise. The clinician may also advise that the individual schedule regular dental checkups, and brush and floss on a daily basis.

Counseling for the 25 to 64-year age population

For the 25 to 64-year age population, counseling should be available or provided in the following areas: substance use, diet and exercise, injury prevention, and sexual behavior. Regarding substance abuse, the patient should be commended for not smoking, or, if the patient does smoke, he or she should be advised to stop smoking. The clinician should provide the smoker with some smoking cessation tips. The patient should also be advised of the ill effects of excessive alcohol use, as well as the dangers of drinking and driving. The importance of a proper, balanced diet and regular physical activity should be stressed as well. Injury prevention includes advising the patient to wear a safety belt, keep weapons in a safe place, and check smoke detectors regularly. Ways to prevent sexually transmitted disease and pregnancy can also be discussed during an intervention.

Counseling for the population older than 65 years of age

Recommended counseling for the population older than 65 is largely similar to that of the 25 to 64-year age population (advice regarding smoking cessation, excess alcohol abuse, diet and exercise, and sexual behavior). However, some additions should be noted regarding injury prevention, as this age group is at greater risk for injury. The standard counseling regarding seat belts, helmets, and smoke detectors is recommended; the clinician should also advise family members of the patient to become CPR certified in case of emergency. The patient (and his or her family members) should be counseled regarding fall prevention (confining the patient to one floor of the house, making sure that the stairs are free of clutter, placing hand rails in the bathroom).

Counseling a couple regarding lifestyle modifications

In some situations, the clinician may find him or herself counseling a patient to stop smoking, eat healthier, and begin an exercise routine, because the patient has developed a number of health problems related to these areas. The clinician may find the patient receptive, but notices that there is no change in behavior from one visit to the next. In this case, it may be beneficial for the clinician to speak to the patient and his or her spouse. Perhaps the patient has good intentions, but has a spouse that enables him or her, or is not supportive of their lifestyle change, and so the patient does not change. By speaking to both the patient and the spouse together, the clinician may be able to get both to realize the importance of changing their habits. By committing to a change together, they may have a greater chance of succeeding.

Pender's Health Promotion Model

Pender developed the Health Promotion Model in an effort to educate APRNs and other clinicians about the psychosocial aspects of health promotion behavior. Her model theorizes that an individual's tendency toward health-promoting behavior is affected by his or her previous behavior, as well as his or her inherited and acquired behavioral characteristics. The individual will commit to changing his or her behavior if he or she values the benefits gained from doing so; conversely, if the individual perceives barriers in achieving these benefits, commitment may waver, and behavior modification may be abandoned. An important barrier between current behavior and behavior modification is whether the individual believes that he or she actually can accomplish an effective change in behavior with expected results.

Health policy

Health policy – Movement in the direction of primary medical attention and getting prevention earlier; encourages utilization of APRNs. The main elements that control healthcare delivery are payors, insurance companies, providers, and suppliers. Legislation regarding ways to do things and politics is included in this topic.

Medical attention – May be primary health care or managed care. Managed care includes Health Maintenance Organizations (HMO), Preferred Provider Organizations (PPO) and Point of Service (POS) plans.

HIPAA privacy directive

HIPAA – Health Insurance Portability and Accountability Act of 1996, under Public Law 104-191. This has a goal of better organization and helpfulness in the medical system, which is to be done by regulating the way that electronic communications for administrative and economic information is done. The requirements include particular transaction regulations (including code sets), security and electronic signatures, privacy and particular identifiers that also have utilization permissions for bosses, health plans and people who give medical attention.

HIPAA privacy – Privacy directives manage how patient's Protected Health Information (PHI) is utilized and given out for times when the data might reveal who the patient is. HIPAA controlled PHI for people who work in the health profession, health plans and health care clearing houses. The aim is to give tough Federal shields for the right to privacy and keep the best medical attention possible. All data is protected. Under this rule, there is a covered entity including the people who do the medical attention that communicate data electronically (as in billing, claims, or paying issues), health plans, and health care clearinghouses. Utilization and giving out of the protected information has to be done to the patient when he asks for it, to HHS, or to check up on or find out if the rule is being complied to. It is allowed for the patient, treatment, payment and healthcare operations (TPO), with the chance to concur or not, public policy, "incident to", restricted information set, and with permission.

HIPAA individual rights:
- Covered entity duties and contact name, title, or telephone to take delivery of grievances with effectual month, day, and year.
- Access, with the right to look at and get a copy of PHI in a designated record set (DRS) in an appropriate time frame.
- Amendment, so that each patient has the right for Covered Entity amend PHI, but this can be not approved by Covered Entity even when the account is correct and finished.
- Accounting, so that the patient has the right to get a record of what information was given out from PHI for 6 years (or less) before the month, day and year that it was asked for.
- Asked for restrictions, so that the patient can ask for limitations of utilization and giving out PHI (although Covered Entity may not allow).
- Confidential communication, so that the provider has to allow and accommodate justifiable desires for PHI information that was exchanged by alternative methods and to alternative places.
- Grievances to covered Entity.
- Grievances to Secretary (HHS/OCR).

Deidentification of PHI for HIPAA

De-identification of PHI – Taking out particular identifiers makes it so the patient cannot be known; use of statistical technique or taking out listed identifiers (like name, geography, dates, or SSN).

Administrative necessities – Put into practice standard ways of doing things with regard to PHI that will go along with the Privacy Rule, put into practice suitable ways to maintain privacy of PHI for administrative, technical, and physical matters, make sure there is privacy education for anyone that is employed there and make and use a way to penalize anyone that does not go along with the Privacy Rule, and select someone to be formally responsible for the standards and ways of doing things and for taking any grievances. The Privacy Rule was obligatory from April 14, 2003. The Office for Civil Rights (OCR) implements it.

Grievances – An unceremonious assessment might give resolution to the problem in total with no official assessment becoming necessary. When it does not, start the official queries. Technical help is available.

Civil Monetary Penalties with regard to HIPAA

Civil Monetary Penalties (CMP) – It is $100 for each infringement. The most one would have to pay is $25,000 for one calendar year for every like condition or prohibition that is infringed upon. It is a criminal penalty for unlawfully giving out information, with these consequences:
- Up to $50,000 plus a year of jail time;.
- Up to $100,000 plus 5 years of jail time for information given out with false pretenses.
- Up to $250,000 plus 10 years of jail time for plan to sell, transfer, or utilize the data for commercial reasons, own gain, or malevolent reasons.
- These consequences are maintained by the Department of Justice (DOJ).

ERISA – Federal law that excuses self-funded medical and additional benefit packages (employer and union) from State authority. Seven of every 10 workers in the United States are in self-insured packages. Official disputes are being done in opposition to the extent of these ERISA exceptions.

Ethics of care

The ethics of care, or the ethical theory of caring, is considered a normative ethical theory, meaning that the theory is based on what individuals should believe is right, instead of what individuals do believe is right. Normative ethical theories examine why certain actions are right or wrong, and why people believe that they are right or wrong, instead of adhering to strict rules about rightness and wrongness. The ethical theory of caring was proposed by feminists who felt that most traditional ethical theories were based on a male approach to problems; justice and impartiality were the guiding forces in ethical decisions. The ethical theory of caring addresses the issue that human relationships introduce complexities into ethical situations, and, as such, universal, impartial ethical rules are not sufficient bases for complex situations.

Deontological theory of ethics

Individuals who follow the deontological theory of ethics operate under the moral belief that ethical decisions should be made based on whether the action is right or wrong, and not on whether the consequences of the actions are right or wrong. Within the area of deontological ethics, however, there are those who believe that there are some actions, though not normally considered to be ethically right, that are justified based on the outcome; for example, lying is wrong, but if the consequence of the lie is that someone's life will be saved, then the lie may be seen as acceptable. Other deontologists (Kantian deontologists, named for Immanuel Kant) follow what is called moral absolutism, meaning that they will always base actions on whether the action is right, regardless of the consequences.

Principle-based theory of ethics

Individuals who follow principle-based theory of ethics are guided by a set of rules, or principles, to make ethical decisions. The rules and principles that constitute principle-based ethics are formed using common and generally accepted moral practices and ideals. The principles are grouped into 4 general categories: respect for autonomy, beneficence, nonmaleficence, and justice. These 4 categories of principles share the following 2 characteristics: they are universal, meaning that they can be applied to all situations in all cultural groups; and they are all prima facie ("first appearance") binding, which means that they are accepted as the preferred method, although there may be situations in which the principle is trumped by a stronger moral consideration.

Virtue ethics

Virtue ethics is a branch of ethics that is much different than utilitarian ethics and deontological ethics. Instead of placing importance on rules and outcomes as a basis for ethical decision making, virtue ethics focuses on the character of the individual. The individual is reliant, then, on his or her own character as an ethical guide. An individual who follows virtue ethics can then be described based on his or her "moral character"; that is, his or her moral choices will reflect upon his or her character.

The casuistic theory of ethics is an applied ethical process in which decisions are made on a case-by-case basis using logic and reasoning. Cases can be compared with similar cases to guide ethical decisions.

Utilitarian theory of ethics

The utilitarian theory of ethics (also referred to as the consequentialist theory) is based on the idea that the moral worth of an action is based on the overall utility, or goodness, of its consequence or consequences. Under the utilitarian theory, the ultimate importance of action is the pleasure and happiness that it produces. There are 2 basic types of utilitarianism: act utilitarianism, and rule utilitarianism. Under act utilitarianism, the individual will make his or her decisions based on the amount of pleasure derived; this is the moral code of the act utilitarian. Rule utilitarians, on the other hand, look at all the outcomes of following a particular rule when making an ethical decision. If the rule produces good results more often than it produces bad results, the rule utilitarian will always follow that rule, whereas the act utilitarian will make the decision based on whether following the rule will have a good outcome in that particular instance.

Ethical sensitivity and moral reasoning

Ethics and ethical decision making are an important part of the role of the APRN. The advent of new technology, as well as the boom in medical research, means that the moral road is more difficult for the APRN to navigate. Ethical sensitivity and moral reasoning are vital to the ethical decision-making process. Ethical sensitivity refers to an individual's awareness of the various moral aspects of a situation; because everyone has different values and moral guidelines, ethical sensitivity is different from one person to the next. Moral reasoning is a more analytical approach to an ethical dilemma; it refers to the process of examining all sides of a situation, and then determining what is the most ethical route or choice.

Ethical issues related to treatment of terminally ill patients

There are a number of ethical concerns that healthcare providers and families must face when determining the treatments that are necessary and appropriate for a terminally-ill patient. It is the nurse's responsibility to provide support and information to help parents/families make informed decisions:
- Analgesia - Provide comfort. Ease the dying process.
- Increase sedation and decrease cognition and interaction with family.
- Side effects. May hasten death.
- Active treatments (such as antibiotics, chemotherapy) - Prolong life. Relieve symptoms. Reassure family.
- Prolong the dying process. Side effects may be severe (as with chemotherapy).
- Supplemental nutrition - Relieve family's anxiety that patient is hungry. Prolong life.
- May cause nausea, vomiting. May increase tumor growth with cancer. May increase discomfort.
- IV fluids for hydration - Relieve family's anxiety that patient is thirsty. Keep mouth moist.
- May result in congestive heart failure and pulmonary edema with increased dyspnea. Increased urinary output and incontinence may cause skin breakdown. Prolong dying process.
- Resuscitation efforts - Allow family to deny death is imminent.Cause unnecessary suffering and prolong dying process.

Resolving ethical conflicts

In the health care setting, it is important that ethical conflicts be resolved without harming the patient or compromising care. There are several factors that will affect the course and outcome of an ethical conflict. First, the level of commitment the clinician has to the patient will determine the amount of effort put forth in resolving an ethical conflict. Second, the degree of moral certainty the clinician has will determine the approach to resolution; if the clinician feels that he or she is correct, he or she will most likely not waver in the decision. Third, the amount of time available for resolution is important; if the clinician is pressed for time, he or she will most likely come to a decision faster than if there is not a time constraint, in which case avoidance may occur. Fourth is the cost-benefit ratio; if the patient refuses to negotiate a certain point, for example, it is not worth the time to the clinician to try to influence the patient's decision.

Beneficence

Beneficence is a guiding principle in which an action is performed in such a way that it is beneficial to another person or persons; this is especially important in the world of health care, as the patient is and should always be viewed as a priority. Of course, this can become tricky when a clinician is caring for multiple patients at once, as is often the case; making decisions that constantly benefit one patient to the exclusion of others is a problem, and a compromise of time and resources must be reached. There are 5 basic rules of beneficence: protect the rights of others, prevent harm, remove sources of evil or harm, help individuals with disabilities, and help others in dangerous situations.

Respect for autonomy

Respect for autonomy is one of the four principles that constitute principle-based ethics; it means that people should recognize and respect that each individual has a right to make his or her own choices and formulate his or her own opinions. The individual will make decisions and form opinions based on his or her own guiding values and principles. There are exceptions to the principle of autonomy, however, and these occur when the individual is not capable, for whatever reason, of making his or her own decisions. In these cases (which must be evaluated with care), the respect for autonomy may be trumped in the interest of safety for the individual. Typically, the individual will have an appointed family member or caretaker who will be in charge of making decisions in the instance that the individual cannot.

Moral justification

Because all principles of principle-based ethics are considered prima facie binding, there are many situations in which one principle will be trumped by another principle; this is especially true when applying principle-based ethics to medicine. When a clinician is faced with a decision in which either act may either benefit or potentially harm the patient, he or she must justify the act with the following 4 conditions: first, the act itself must be either morally good or morally neutral; second, the clinician is performing the act with only good intentions, even if he or she can foresee possible ill effects; third, the possible ill effect or effects cannot be prelude or means to the intended good effect; and fourth, the good effect or outcome must outweigh any possible ill effects.

Nonmalfeasance

Nonmalfeasance, another of the 4 guiding principles of principle-based ethics, is the ethical or moral responsibility to avoid intentionally harming another individual. Intentional harm includes disabling or killing another individual, or inflicting pain upon another individual. This is another somewhat tricky principle to apply to medicine, and one can see how prima facie binding applies. For example, a patient is seen in the emergency department for appendicitis; he is in a great deal of pain, and at risk for rupture, peritonitis, and even death without prompt treatment. Surgical removal of the appendix is indicated, which introduces the patient to other risks (scar from surgical procedure, postoperative pain, infection, even death). In cases such as this, nonmalfeasance may be trumped by the principle of beneficence, because the proposed risks are considered to be outweighed by the benefits.

Justice

Justice is an ethical principle that guides individuals to make decisions that are both fair and equal. Distributive justice is a specific theory that focuses on fair and equal treatment of others in regards to distributing goods and services; this theory of justice is easily applicable to medicine and health care. Because a clinician often has a group of patients that he or she is caring for at one time, it is important that the clinician divide supplies, time, and attention between the patients fairly. There are 5 material principles of distributive justice: 1) each person should receive an equal share of goods and/or services; 2) goods and services should be distributed to each individual according to the needs of the individual (entitlement); 3) each individual should receive goods and services according to effort and to 4) contribution and 5) merit.

Distributive justice

To understand how distributive justice applies to medicine, think about a situation in which there are 2 trauma patients in the emergency department. Both patients have lost a lot of blood and are in need of transfusion. The problem is, there are only 6 units of blood available. Who should get the blood? If one patient arrived before the other, should he be entitled? Perhaps he should, but there are other factors to consider. If he is in worse shape than the other patient (in other words, he needs the blood more urgently), than distributive justice would suggest that he should receive the blood. On the other hand, if both patients are in the same relative condition, how should the decision be made? You could look at contribution; if both patients were in a motor vehicle accident, but one was a drunk driver and the other an innocent motorist, it may be acceptable to give the blood to the innocent motorist in a situation where supplies are scarce.

Conflict resolution

There are many ways to attempt conflict resolution, some of them beneficial, some of them not. Avoidance is a strategy that is not typically considered to be beneficial to conflict resolution; when the clinician is not committed to the relationship with the patient, or if the situation is nonemergent, the clinician may ignore or deny the conflict in an effort to avoid facing it. Coercion is another strategy that does not usually end in a favorable outcome, at least for one of the parties involved. This strategy is used when the clinician feels that he or she is right, does not have time to devote to proper resolution, and has not invested time into a relationship with the patient. Accommodation is a somewhat similar strategy, albeit with less resistance, where one party concedes that the other's position is right. Compromise and collaboration are usually the best methods of resolution, and allow both sides to be heard.

Warning signs that might indicate abuse and/or neglect

Regular screening for domestic violence in a healthcare setting is a helpful and inoffensive method of identifying victims. Watch for injuries that do not seem to match the story given. Overbearing or overprotective partners who answer for or dominate your interview with the patient, frequent nonspecific complaints such as headache, stomach, neck and back pain, insecurity, stammering or avoidance in giving responses to simple questions, intestinal complaints, and sexually transmitted disease. In the abused adolescent female tobacco, alcohol and drug use, decreased school attendance, isolation, and bulimia are more common.

The different types of elder abuse include physical, sexual, emotional, financial and neglect. The most likely perpetrator is a family member. Institutional caregivers are also potential abusers of the elderly. Female seniors older than 80 are more likely to be abused. The more dependent an elderly individual is, the greater the chances there are of abuse. Signs of abuse include unexplained cuts, bruises, burns or other injuries. Weight loss, poor hygiene and other unmet needs are also signs there may be neglect, which is a form of abuse. Improper management of valuables and finances should also lead to suspicion of abuse. Nurse practitioners should routinely question elderly patients about the possibility of abuse and take appropriate action if abuse is suspected.

Patients'/families' rights

Patients' (families') rights in relation to what they should expect from a healthcare organization are outlined in both standards of the Joint Commission and National Committee for Quality Assurance. Rights include:
- Respect for patient, including personal dignity and psychosocial, spiritual, and cultural considerations.
- Response to needs related to access and pain control.
- Ability to make decisions about care, including informed consent, advance directives, and end of life care.
- Procedure for registering complaints or grievances.
- Protection of confidentiality and privacy.
- Freedom from abuse or neglect.
- Protection during research and information related to ethical issues of research.
- Appraisal of outcomes, including unexpected outcomes.
- Information about organization, services, and practitioners.
- Appeal procedures for decisions regarding benefits and quality of care.
- Organizational code of ethical behavior.
- Procedures for donating and procuring organs/tissue.

Patient advocacy

Patient advocacy is defined as the process of speaking on behalf of a patient to ensure that his or her rights are protected, and that he or she is provided with necessary information and services. The APRN frequently serves as patient advocate, although physicians, social workers, and other individuals in the health care industry may act on behalf of the patient as well.

The ANA defines nursing as "the protection, promotion, and optimization of health and abilities, prevention of illness and injury, alleviation of suffering through the diagnosis and treatment of human response, and advocacy in the care of individuals, families, communities, and populations."

When a APRN notices that a patient is receiving improper treatment at the hands of another health care worker, be it another APRN, a physician, a social worker, or anyone else who contributes to patient care, he or she may be hesitant to report the improper treatment; this is especially true if the abusive health care worker holds a position of authority over the APRN. Although the APRN may feel that he or she should not report certain instances (even though he or she is aware that the patient is being maltreated), it is important that he or she is aware that this falls under the role of the patient advocate. Ensuring proper treatment of the patient is an important part of the APRN's job, and he or she should not worry about being reprimanded for reporting abuse.

Perhaps the greatest facilitator of patient advocacy is the APRN-patient relationship; if a strong relationship exists between the APRN and the patient, the APRN will be motivated to perform the duties of advocate. If the patient and APRN have a strained or limited relationship, advocacy can be difficult. Recognizing the patient's needs is another facilitator, one that goes hand in hand with a good APRN-patient relationship. If the APRN feels a sense of responsibility and accountability on behalf of the patient, he or she is more likely to serve as a good patient advocate; conscience is a strong motivator. Another facilitator is if the physician acts as a colleague, instead of a superior; this strengthens the APRN-physician relationship, and the APRN feels that he or she can question the physician's judgment instead of constantly deferring. That being said, the greater the knowledge base and skill level of the APRN, the greater he or she will be as an advocate.

Informed consent

Patients or guardians must provide informed consent for all treatment the patient receives. This includes a thorough explanation of all procedures and treatment and associated risks. Patients/guardians should be apprised of all options and allowed input on the type of treatments. Patients/guardians should be apprised of all reasonable risks and any complications that might be life threatening or increase morbidity. The American Medical Association has established guidelines for informed consent:
- Explanation of diagnosis.
- Nature and reason for treatment or procedure.
- Risks and benefits.
- Alternative options (regardless of cost or insurance coverage).
- Risks and benefits of alternative options.
- Risks and benefits of not having a treatment or procedure.

Providing informed consent is a requirement of all states.

Competency

Competency of the geriatric patient is generally determined by state law. Four principles define competency:
1. A patient must be able to understand his/her situation and the potential consequences.
2. He/she must be able to understand all relevant information.
3. He/she must be able to process that information in a rational manner.
4. He/she must be able to communicate his/her wishes in a coherent manner.

When there is a question of competency and a conflict between the wishes of the patient and the family's wishes, a competency evaluation may be needed. In general, a court will appoint a psychiatrist to evaluate the patient, but the decision about competency is made by a judge. If a patient is determined to be incompetent, the court will appoint a guardian for the patient. This guardian then has legal decision-making power over the healthcare decisions for the patient called a durable Power of Attorney.

Advance care planning

Advance care planning is the process of planning for potential medical situations or crises that would impact a person's health or disability. It involves considering potential situations that could occur before they actually happen and then making plans for what to do in case those situations were to occur. Advance care planning gives people security about health care in the future, in case they are unable to make medical decisions for themselves. An example of advance care planning is to develop an advance directive, which guides clinicians as to the types of treatments the patient would like if he/she became unable to make those decisions. Advance care planning may also involve appointing a power of attorney to make legal decisions regarding medical care. Taking steps to plan for potential problems through advance care planning provides peace of mind for people to face the future with possible health problems.

Advance care planning outlines the desires of the patient and has been planned in advance. If the patient is unable to make decisions, the advanced care plan speaks the wishes of the patient. Nurse practitioners can play a crucial role in helping patients with advance care planning by beginning the conversation with a patient about whether or not they have an advance care plan in place, and guiding the patient on steps to create one if the patient does not have one. The nurse practitioner should be available to explain disease processes and expectations regarding symptoms and pain that could occur based on the patient's condition, as well as procedure options and their ability to prolong life. The nurse practitioner can also explain what types of care can be provided in different settings and answer questions about quality at the end of life. It is also the nurse practitioner's responsibility to be aware of what type of advance care planning a patient has in place, especially if the patient has a terminal or chronic disease. If something were to happen, the nurse practitioner's awareness of the patient's wishes will guide her decision making for the patient's care. Finally, when applicable, the nurse practitioner can use the patient's advanced care planning to write orders for the patient that hospital personnel can actually follow, such as translating an advanced directive that states the patient does not want CPR into an actual Do Not Resuscitate Order.

Theory-practice gap

The theory-practice gap refers to the lack of communication between researchers and clinicians; while researchers are working to develop new treatments and methodologies, clinicians are busy treating patients and may not have the time to educate themselves about what is new in the research world. On the other side, the research community is probably not familiar with the clinical applications of the current methodologies. It is important for both sides to take an active role in communicating with one another in an effort to bridge the gap; active communication between researchers and clinicians can help disseminate new research ideas and methods into practice, and can educate researchers about what will and will not work in the clinical setting.

The theory-practice gap exists because clinicians and researchers traditionally work in 2 separate worlds; the clinical community is directly involved in patient care on a daily basis, while the research community is removed from the realm of patient care. Both communities, however, have the same goal, and that is to improve patient care and quality of life. Establishing communication and camaraderie between the 2 communities is incredibly beneficial for both sides. Training sessions in which clinicians are educated about research practices and researchers are trained about clinical practices are a good start. Facilitating research collaborations between researchers and clinicians is another great way to improve communication. Clinician-researchers can function as intermediaries between the 2 communities, and can educate others. The development of standard operating procedures or best practice guidelines for the transfer of knowledge is also important.

Institutional Theory

Institutional Theory (IT), generally defined, is a theory based on the idea that it is difficult to develop institution-wide rules because there are individuals within the institution to whom the rules may not apply. These generalized institutional rules may not be feasible when applied to the daily practice of the individuals operating within the institution. This results in a gap between the actual rules of the organization and what is done by the individuals within; if the rules are not feasible, the individual may engage in evidence-based decision making. This gap between the rules and the shift to evidence-based decision making will make it more difficult to transfer knowledge both within the clinical community and between the research community and the clinical community.

Clinical study

Clinical challenging and other scientific-based questioning of clinical practice will often lead to questions about clinical care that the clinician does not have answers to. In these cases, the clinician may decide to develop a clinical study with the goal of answering the specific clinical question. When the clinician decides that he or she is interested in developing a research project, there are important steps that need to be followed, and important questions that need to be asked. First and foremost, the clinician needs to ask him or herself whether the study is feasible. In other words, can the study be accomplished in a reasonable amount of time, without enlisting the help of numerous people? The clinician also needs to understand all of the elements that must be included in the project, including the exact research methods, the importance of having informed consent from the patients involved in the study, the cost, and various other aspects.

Study design

When the APRN decides that he or she wishes to conduct a case study or a set of case studies for research purposes, he or she must design the case study in such a way that he or she elicits the most information possible from the study. First, the APRN must decide what research question or questions he or she aims to answer by conducting the case study. Second, the APRN must identify the proposition or propositions of the study. Third, the APRN must determine what exactly he or she wishes to analyze in the case study; that is, what components are vital to the questions that need to be answered. Fourth, the APRN must determine how he or she will link the data gathered through the case study to the proposition(s) of the study. Fifth, the APRN must develop standard criteria to interpret the findings yielded by the study.

Evidence-based practice

Evidence-based practice – Meticulous, well-judged, and precise utilization of recent most excellent proof regarding medical attention for each patient that uses both medical know-how and patient ideals. The main types of primary research include:
- Therapy – To assess how well the medical attention is going. Random, double-blind, placebo-managed.
- Identification of conditions and screening – Takes accounts of legitimacy and dependability for assessments or assesses how well the assessment works to identify a condition before patient indications occur. Cross-sectional survey.
- Causation or harm – Checks if a substance is linked to an arising health problem. Cohort or case-managed.
- Prognosis – Predicts how the condition will turn out. Longitudinal cohort study.
- Systemic review – Synopsis of published works which utilizes particular ways to work to do a complete published works investigation and critical evaluation of particular studies; utilizes proper statistics to put the legitimate studies together.
- Meta-analysis – Methodical review; quantitative. Makes a synopsis of outcome.

Levels of strength of evidence-based practice:
- Level I (A–D) – Meta-analysis or a number of controlled studies together.
- Level II (A–D) – Individual experimental study.
- Level III (A–D) – Quasi-experimental study.
- Level IV (A–D) – Nonexperimental study.
- Level V (A–D) – Case report or methodically acquired; confirmable quality or program assessment information.
- Level VI – Judgment of esteemed authorities; also regulatory or legal opinions.

Prevention – courses of action are published in:

Put Prevention into Practice – U.S. Public Health Service; regarding prevention for primary medical attention.

Clinicians Handbook of Preventive Service: Put Prevention Into Practice, 1998 – for primary medical attention; http://www.ahcpr.gov/clinic/ppiphand.htm.

Guide to Clinical Preventive Services, U.S. Preventive Services Task Force, 1996 – for both practice and instructional atmospheres.

Statistics

Statistics – It is important to be able to comprehend research that has been done to improve medical practices in a clinical setting. It is important for the reader to be able to read the data and comprehend how much worth the study has for his or her particular situation. Since the study might not give the complete scope of what was discovered and another person's analysis of it may be based on a particular point of view that is not relevant to the nurse, the nurse needs to be able to read and understand research reports. If the nurse reads a research report that does not include statistics, it still is not a frittered time because it could bring up new matter about best practices.

Pearson's correlation – Also called Pearson product-moment correlation coefficient (PMCC); common way to measure the relationship between two (or more) variables. It actually identifies the relationship.

Factor analysis – Utilized for finding common elements between variables.

Research

Research is an important part of patient care because medical advances made possible through research are the basis of future treatment modalities and care plans. The APRN, as an advanced practice nurse, is in the perfect position to facilitate research and coordinate research efforts with current clinical practice. However, because the professional role of the APRN is extensive, and because patient care is the most important part of the APRN's role, it is difficult for the APRN to find time to devote to research opportunities; it is especially difficult because there is no clearly defined research role for the APRN. There are opportunities for APRNs to work in a more research-oriented environment, and they can contribute a great deal to research efforts. APRNs who work in clinical settings (as most do) may find it difficult to devote time to research.

Nurses, nurse practitioners, physicians, and other clinicians are often too busy to devote time to exploring the latest research advances, which could potentially be used to institute a change in practice that would greatly benefit patients. Reviewing literature can be a tedious and time-consuming process that just does not fit into the schedule of the busy clinician. There are ways that clinicians can find information about the latest practice changes and new guidelines; organizations like the Centers for Disease Control and Prevention (CDC), the National Institutes of Health (NIH), the National Cancer Institute (NCI), and the AACN often provide this information. These organizations review the literature and develop best practices, research-based protocols, and guidelines for clinicians to follow when instituting practice changes.

Research for advanced practice

Research for advanced practice – Utilized for creating new research; founded clinical ways of working, to keep a record of clinical results and differences, to show excellence and ways to keep expenses down for medical attention, to create organization for demonstration tasks, and to get more excellent care and better results for the patient. For the patient, research is a good thing because it gives a better comprehension of the patient's circumstances, gives a better evaluation of the circumstances, results in more value in the medical treatment, creates a situation of more understanding for the patient's circumstance, and helps providers better identify the requirement for and success of treatment plans. The problems include time and expense, workers that do not want to make alterations, no rewards for utilizing the results of the study, and incomprehension or doubt about the research results. To deal with these problems, make an atmosphere that sees the use of and will utilize the study, make an atmosphere that encourages inquiry, rational thought and assesses nursing care, and promote research by giving enough time and money for it.

Research for advanced practice – Research founded on practice is vital for getting better advanced practice nursing for years to come. The most important drift these days is toward outcome studies. You may find outcomes of studies at conferences, in publications, or through summaries of the studies themselves. Research may be paid for by the federal government, including:

- Agency for Healthcare Research and Quality (AHRQ) – http://www.ahcpr.gov
- National Institutes of Health (NIH) – http://www.nih.gov
- Maternal and Child Health Bureau (MCHB) – http://www.mchb.hrsa.gov

Patient consent for research

Patient consent – If you are doing research that has patients involved, the most vital piece to include is the assertion that everything will be private and confidential. This piece is necessary and it is against the law to leave it out.

New research – Use a new practice based on research in a clinical setting if the outcome of the research showed statistically significant results. It is hard in ambulatory care environments because the job is so challenging that there is not much time left for using new research. Lack of time is a factor in every medical care environment. Getting the research is not usually the problem since it can be acquired through the internet or in professional journals. Quite a bit of research has been done regarding ambulatory care environments. Using new research in a clinical setting commonly has the outcome of an alteration in the way things are done. Nursing is a lot like research.

Qualitative nursing research

Qualitative nursing research – The aim is to find and describe concepts of nursing. It does not include exact measurements and does not generally include statistics.

Standard deviation – Measures the dispersion of data; it is the square root of variance.

Example: the regular ranges for blood work values would probably be put in a standard deviation as a statistic.

Steps to using research:
- Find the problems.
- Evaluate published work.
- Create the new idea.
- Assess.
- Determine if you will use the new idea.

Healthcare practice – Is in the middle of changes due to the Patient Protection and Affordable Care Act. This regulatory overhaul of the current healthcare system was signed into law in 2010, but the extent of all the changes has yet to be seen, as all provisions will be slowly phased in over time until the year 2020.

Case study methodology

A great method of gaining information <u>for</u> the APRN is through case study methodology. The definition of a case study is "a systematic inquiry into an event or set of related events which aims to describe and explain the phenomenon of interest" (Bromley). The APRN, who has a great deal of interaction with the patient, will find that case studies are a great resource for information. When conducting a case study, the APRN will conduct a complete, comprehensive, in-depth interview of the patient, review the patient's medical records, and observe the patient.

Resource-Based View

The Resource-Based View (RBV) is a theory first developed by economists with the purpose of determining the resources available to a firm or institution. It is an organizational study of the effectiveness of an institution as a result of the resources available to the institution. When applied to the theory-practice gap, the RBV is that the transfer of knowledge within and between organizations or institutions (in this case, between the clinical setting and the research setting) is costly and difficult, based on the fact that the capacity of the clinical community to absorb knowledge is low. To correct for this, the RBV states that available resources should be used to enhance and expand the learning and absorptive capacity of the clinical community.

Changes in methodology that are not always based on true research

The nurse practitioner is assuming an increasingly autonomous role as a health care provider because an emphasis is placed on the nurse practitioner being an "advanced practice" clinician. The nurse practitioner may find him or herself managing a clinic with a high patient volume, or he or she may be considered an equal to resident physicians as far as responsibilities are concerned. Nurse practitioners find that they are given more patient-management responsibilities, and do not have time for teaching, education, and research. This can lead to the nurse practitioner making clinical decisions based on results that he or she observes in the clinical setting ("consensus-based" practice) instead of making decisions based on results gained from actual research-based practice.

Resistance to organizational change

Performance improvement processes cannot occur without organizational change, and resistance to change is common for many people, so coordinating collaborative processes requires anticipating resistance and taking steps to achieve cooperation. Resistance often relates to concerns about job loss, increased responsibilities, and general denial or lack of understanding and frustration. Leaders can prepare others involved in the process of change by taking these steps:
- Be honest, informative, and tactful, giving people thorough information about anticipated changes and how the changes will affect them, including positives.
- Be patient in allowing people the time they need to contemplate changes and express anger or disagreement.
- Be empathetic in listening carefully to the concerns of others.
- Encourage participation, allowing staff to propose methods of implementing change, so they feel some sense of ownership.

- Establish a climate in which all staff members are encouraged to identify the need for change on an ongoing basis.
- Present further ideas for change to management.

Gathering meaning from research data

The data gathered from studies are often diverse, and it can be difficult to determine what is important and what is not. To determine whether data are meaningful, there are some strategies that the APRN can use. First, the APRN can look at the data to determine whether there are any patterns to see which data go with which. Then, the APRN should aim to increase his or her understanding of the data; this can be done by making comparisons between data sets, and by separating different variables within the data sets. Next, the APRN can inspect the data to see if there are any relationships between variables. Once the data have been examined and sorted, the APRN can assemble the data coherently by building a logical chain linking data and variables.

Independent Practice

Health assessment

Health assessment – Get an account of prior health issues so that you will know what activities give the patient more of a chance of problems and you will be able to give the proper instruction for that patient. The health history should include demographics and biographical information. It should include an account of current health problems, including the OPQRST assessment:
- Onset
- Provocative/palliative (getting well or problem going downhill)
- Quality/quantity
- Region/radiation
- Setting
- Timing

Find out about prior health issues, including how the patient feels he is generally doing, prior conditions or times in the hospital, harm or operations (including when, what the medical attention was, and what check-ups were done afterwards), emotional well-being, sexual well-being, allergies to food or drugs (and the particular problem that happens including needed medical attention for it if there is any), drugs (prescribed and over-the-counter), immunizations (when and what), sleep routines, and prior assessments for any part of the body. Discuss individual routines, including the utilization of tobacco, alcohol, drugs, caffeine, nutrition, physical activity, hobbies, athletics, and contact sports.

Confusion Assessment Method

The Confusion Assessment Method is used to assess the development of delirium and is intended for those without psychiatric training. The tool covers 9 factors. Some factors have a range of possibilities and others are rated only as to whether the characteristic is present, not present, uncertain, or not applicable. The tool provides room to describe abnormal behavior. Factors indicative of delirium include:
- Onset: Acute change in mental status.
- Attention: Inattentive, stable or fluctuating.
- Thinking: Disorganized, rambling conversation, switching topics, illogical,
- Level of consciousness: Altered, ranging from alert to coma.
- Orientation: Disoriented (person, place, time)
- Memory: Impaired.
- Perceptual disturbances: Hallucinations, illusions.
- Psychomotor abnormalities: Agitation (tapping, picking, moving) or retardation (staring, not moving).
- Sleep-wake cycle: Awake at night and sleepy in the daytime.

The tool indicates delirium if there is an acute onset with fluctuating inattention and disorganized thinking or altered level of consciousness.

Cognitive assessment

Individuals with evidence of dementia or short-term memory loss, often associated with Alzheimer's disease, should have cognition assessed. The Mini-mental state exam (MMSE) or the Mini-cog test is commonly used. Both require the individual to carry out specified tasks.

MMSE:
- Remembering and later repeating the names of 3 common objects.
- Counting backward from 100 by 7s or spelling "world" backward.
- Naming items as the examiner points to them.
- Providing the location of the examiner's office, including city, state, and street address.
- Repeating common phrases.
- Copying a picture of interlocking shapes.
- Following simple 3-part instructions, such a picking up a piece of paper, folding it in half, and placing it on the floor.

A score of $\geq 24/30$ is considered a normal functioning level.

Mini-cog:
- Remembering and later repeating the names of 3 common objects.
- Drawing the face of a clock with all 12 numbers and the hands indicating the time specified by the examiner.

Administration of medication

It is extremely important that the utmost care be taken when administering medication; administering the incorrect medication, the wrong dosage, or a medication to which the patient is allergic can have disastrous consequences. A helpful way to make sure that all the bases are covered is to remember the "rights" of medication administration. First, the APRN should check to make sure that he or she has the right patient. Next, the APRN should make sure that he or she is administering the right medication. Then, the APRN should check to make sure that the dosage is correct. Making sure that the route of administration is correct is also important. Next, the APRN should make sure that the medication is being administered at the correct time. Finally, the APRN should make sure that the documentation regarding the medication administration is correct.

Basic patient safety assessments

There are 4 basic assessments that the APRN should make when assessing a patient's safety and identifying possible safety concerns. The first of these is the mobility assessment; different safety risks apply to patients who are mobile as opposed to those who are not. An immobile patient, for example, has a tendency to form pressure ulcers, or bedsores. The next assessment is the evaluation of the patient's level of awareness; is the patient able to communicate to the nursing staff when something is wrong? If not, certain measures should be undertaken to ensure that the nursing staff is aware of a change in the patient's condition. An extension of this assessment is determining whether the patient is in critical condition; these patients must be monitored more closely for changes. An assessment of the patient's mental status is also important, because the patient may not be able to make safe decisions on his or her own.

Functional evaluation of the elderly patient

Functional evaluation of the elderly patient – Get an account of how the patient has been disabled including bodily, emotional, mental and community considerations. Check for sensorimotor function. Find out how the patient is handling the situation. Check thinking and reasoning abilities. Find out if the patient can keep up with his or her place in society.

Problems that can influence the ability to function include sight or hearing problems that come before or make worse the patient's bewilderment, new environment that can create bewilderment or problems with sleeping, musculoskeletal harm that creates a problem with movement, makes the patient more dependent, and causes less control and more problems with sleeping.

Physical evaluation of the elderly patient includes basic examination, regular alterations due to aging, integumentary system, cardiovascular system, respiratory system, breasts, gastrointestinal system, genitourinary and reproductive system, endocrine system, musculoskeletal system, senses, and neurological system. For each, check for anatomical and physiological alterations, clinical connotations, and irregularities or disease.

Activities of daily living

Activities of daily living (ADLs) are a group of activities that are used to evaluate a patient's return to normal function; these are activities that the patient had performed on a daily basis before hospitalization, and will be expected to perform once he or she has completed rehabilitation. The rate at which the patient accomplishes these activities, in addition to the level of independence maintained by the patient when performing the activities, can help caregivers determine the amount of rehabilitation required, and can also be used to monitor the progress of the patient during the rehabilitation process. ADLs are grouped into 3 different areas: personal and physical, instrumental, and occupational.

The first group of ADLs, the physical or personal group, contains those daily activities that relate to the patient's ability to take care of him or herself. Included in this group are activities related to health management, nutritional needs, elimination of bladder and bowel contents, exercise, self-esteem, coping/stress management, cognitive abilities, communication, sexual health and ability, and relationship roles. The second group of ADLs, the instrumental group, contains activities such as shopping, answering the phone, and other activities that involve leaving home. The third group, occupational activities, includes activities that are required of being a parent, husband, or wife, as well as those required on the job.

Information needed for the health history of an elderly patient

Health history of elderly patient – Biographical information, family background regarding medical histories, job, drugs being used, use of cigarettes, use of drugs that are against the law, allergies, problems with drugs or foods, mental problems, diet, sleep, physical activity, leisure activities, overview of systems, and prevention being done (such as screenings). Get an account of the prior medical treatment, including any time the patient had to go to the hospital, surgeries, vaccinations, accidents, harm done, falling down, medical conditions from the past (including as a kid), communicable diseases from the past, health practices, and religious elements that influence the body (such as fasting). Check into safety concerns including work, home, and other places, the ability to drive, or any abuse. Discuss the Patient Self-Determination Act from 1990, including any advance directives, a living will, power of attorney, and doctor-assisted suicide. Find out where and with whom the patient lives, including who the main caregiver is. Talk about how a disability will affect income, and discuss help that can be found in the area.

Myocardial infarction

Diagnosis of a myocardial infraction includes a complete physical examination and patient and family history with assessment of risk factors. Assessment may include:
- ECG obtained immediately to monitor heart changes over time. Typical changes include T-wave inversion, elevation of ST segment, and abnormal Q waves.
- Echocardiogram to evaluate ventricular function.
- Creatine kinase (CK) and isoenzyme (MB):
  o CK-MB (cardiac muscle) level increases within a few hours and peaks at about 24 hours (earlier with thrombolytic therapy or PTCA).
- Myoglobin (heme protein that transports oxygen) found in both skeletal and cardiac muscles. Levels increase in 1-3 hours after an MI and peak within 12 hours. While an increase is not specific to an MI, a failure to increase can be used to rule out an MI.
- Troponin (protein in the myocardium) and its isomers (C, I, and T) regulate contraction and levels increase as with CK-MB, but levels remains elevated for up to 3 weeks.

Intraaortic balloon pump

The intraaortic balloon (IAB) pump is the most commonly used circulatory assist device. It is used for a number of problems:
- After cardiac surgery to treat left ventricular failure.
- Unstable angina.
- Myocardial infarction with complications or persistent angina.
- Cardiogenic shock.
- Papillary muscle dysfunction or rupture with mitral regurgitation or ventricular septal rupture.
- Ventricular dysrhythmias that don't respond to treatment.

The IABP comprises a catheter with an inflatable balloon from the tip and lengthwise down the catheter. The catheter is usually inserted through the femoral artery but may be placed during surgery or through a cutdown. The catheter is threaded into the descending thoracis aorta, and the balloon inflates during diastole to increase circulation to the coronary arteries, and then deflates during systole to decrease afterload. Complications include:
- Dysrhythmias.
- Peripheral ischemia from femoral artery occlusion.
- Balloon perforation or migration.

Percutaneous coronary interventions

Percutaneous transluminal coronary angioplasty (PTCA) is an option for people who are poor surgical candidates, who have an acute MI, or who have uncontrolled chest pain. This procedure is usually only done to increase circulation to the myocardium by breaking through an atheroma if there is collateral circulation. Cardiac catheterization is done with a hollow catheter (sheath), usually inserted into the femoral vein or artery and fed through the vessels to the coronary arteries. When the atheroma is verified by fluoroscopy, a balloon-tipped catheter is fed over the sheath and the balloon is inflated with a contrast agent, to a specified pressure to compress the atheroma. The balloon may be inflated a number of times to ensure that residual stenosis is <20%. Laser angioplasty using the excimer laser is also used to vaporize plaque. **Stents** may be inserted during the angioplasty to maintain patency. Stents may be flexible plastic or wire mesh and are typically placed over the catheter, which is inflated to expand the stent against the arterial wall.

Cardiac catheterization and PTCA

Cardiac catheterization and PTCA poses the risk of both intraoperative and postoperative complications. During the procedure, there is a risk of damage to both the coronary artery and the heart itself. The artery may dissect, perforate, or constrict with vasospasm. A myocardial infarction may occur when a clot dislodges. Ventricular tachycardia or cardiac arrest may occur. These complications may require immediate surgical repair. Postoperative complications of cardiac catheterization/PCTA include:
- Hemorrhage or hematoma at sheath insertion site may require pressure. Head of bed should be flat to relieve pressure.
- Thrombus or embolus may require further surgery and/or anticoagulation/thrombolytic treatment.
- Arteriovenous fistula or pseudoaneurysm from vessel trauma usually requires compression with ultrasound and surgical repair.
- Retroperitoneal bleeding from an arterial tear may cause back or flank pain and may require discontinuation of anticoagulants and IV fluids and/or blood transfusions.
- Failure of angioplasty may require repeat procedure or other surgical intervention.

Preventing complications from ventilators

Methods to prevent complications from mechanical ventilation include:
- Elevate patient's head and chest to 30° to prevent aspiration and ventilation-associated pneumonia.
- Reposition patient every 2 hours.
- Provide DVT prophylaxis, such as external compression support and/or heparin (5000 u sq 2-3 times daily).
- Administer famotidine (20 mg BID per NG tube or IV) or sucralfate (1 gram per NG tube QID) to prevent gastrointestinal bleeding.
- Decrease and eliminate sedation/analgesia as soon as possible.
- Follow careful protocols for pressure settings to prevent barotrauma. Tidal volumes are usually maintained at 8 to 10 mg/kg PBW.
- Monitor for pneumothorax or evidence of barotrauma.
- Conduct nutritional assessment (including lab tests) to prevent malnutrition.

- Monitor intake and output carefully and administer IV fluids to prevent dehydration.
- Do daily spontaneous breathing trials and discontinue ventilation as soon as possible.

Indications for surgical/vascular interventions for arterial insufficiency/ ulcers

The goals of management for arterial insufficiency and ulcers is to improve perfusion and save the limb, but lifestyle changes and medications may be insufficient. There are a number of indications for surgical intervention:
- Poor healing prognosis includes those with ABI < 0.5 because their perfusion is severely compromised.
- Failure to respond to conservative treatment (medications and lifestyle changes) even with an ABI > 0.5.
- Intolerable pain, such as with severe intermittent claudication, which is incapacitating and limits the patient's ability to work or carry out activities. Rest pain is an indication that medical treatment is insufficient.
- Limb-threatening condition, such as severe ischemia with increasing pain at rest, infection, and/or gangrene. Infection can cause a wound to deteriorate rapidly.

Surgical intervention is indicated only for those patients with patent distal vessels as demonstrated by radiologic imaging procedures.

Cardiac dysrhythmias

Cardiac dysrhythmias, abnormal heart beats, in adults are frequently the result of damage to the conduction system during major cardiac surgery or as the result of a myocardial infarction.

Bradydysrhythmia are pulse rates that are abnormally slow:
- Complete atrioventricular block (A-V block) may be congenital or a response to surgical trauma.
- Sinus bradycardia may be caused by the autonomic nervous system or a response to hypotension and decrease in oxygenation.
- Junctional/nodal rhythms often occur in post-surgical patients when absence of P wave is noted but heart rate and output usually remain stable, and unless there is compromise, usually no treatment is necessary.

Tachydysrhythmia are pulse rates that are abnormally fast:
- Sinus tachycardia is often caused by illness, such as fever or infection.
- Supraventricular tachycardia (200-300 bpm) may have a sudden onset and result in congestive heart failure.

Conduction irregularities are irregular pulses that often occur post-operatively and are usually not significant:
- Premature contractions may arise from the atria or ventricles.

Electrocardiogram

The electrocardiogram records and shows a graphic display of the electrical activity of the heart through a number of different waveforms, complexes, and intervals:
- P wave: Start of electrical impulse in the sinus node and spreading through the atria, muscle depolarization.
- QRS complex: Ventricular muscle depolarization and atrial repolarization.
- T wave: Ventricular muscle repolarization (resting state) as cells regain negative charge.
- U wave: Repolarization of the Purkinje fibers.

A modified lead II ECG is often used to monitor basic heart rhythms and dysrhythmias:
- Typical placement of leads for 2-lead ECG is 3 to 5 cm inferior to the right clavicle and left lower ribcage. Typical placement for 3-lead ECG is (RA) right arm near shoulder, (LA) V_5 position over 5th intercostal space, and (LL) left upper leg near groin.

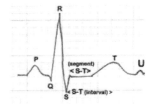

Hemodynamic monitoring and oxygen saturation

Hemodynamic monitoring includes monitoring oxygen saturation levels, which must be maintained for proper cardiac function. Changes in the oxygen saturation levels can indicate complications in the post-surgical patient. The central venous catheter often has an oxygen sensor at the tip to monitor oxygen saturation in the right atrium. If the catheter tip is located near the renal veins, this can cause an increase in right atrial oxygen saturation; and near the coronary sinus, a decrease:
- Increased oxygen saturation may result form left atrial to right atrial shunt, abnormal pulmonary venous return, increased delivery of oxygen or decrease in extraction of oxygen.
- Decreased oxygen saturation may be related to low cardiac output with an increase in oxygen extraction or decrease in arterial oxygen saturation with normal differences in the atrial and ventricular oxygen saturation.

Hemodynamic monitoring and intraarterial blood pressure monitoring

Intraarterial blood pressure monitoring is done for systolic, diastolic, and mean arterial pressure (MAP) for conditions that decrease cardiac output, tissue perfusion, or fluid volume. A catheter is inserted into an artery, such as the radial (most frequently used), dorsalis pedis, femoral, or axillary, percutaneously or through a cut-down. Before catheter insertion, collateral circulation must be assessed by Doppler or the Allen test (used for the hand). In the Allen test, both the radial and ulnar artery are compressed and the patient is asked to clench the hand repeatedly until it blanches, and then one artery is released, and the tissue on that side should flush. Then the test is repeated again, releasing the other artery. The MAP is most commonly used to evaluate perfusion as it shows pressure

- 85 -

throughout the cardiac cycle. Systole is one-third and diastole two-thirds of the normal cardiac cycle. The MAP for a blood pressure of 120/60 (Normal range 70-100 mm Hg):

- $\frac{[(Diastole \times 2) + (Systole \times 1)]}{3}$ = MAP
- $\frac{(60 \times 2 = 120) + (120)}{3}$ = 240 = MAP of 80.

Cardiac output

Cardiac output (CO) is the amount of blood is pumped through the ventricles during a specified period. Normal cardiac output is about 5 liters per minutes at rest for an adult. Under exercise or stress, this volume may multiply 3 or 4 times with concomitant changes in the heart rate (HR) and stroke volume (SV). The basic formulation for calculating cardiac output is the heart rate (HR) per minute multiplied by measurement by the stroke volume (SR), which is the amount of blood pumped through the ventricles with each contraction. The stroke volume is controlled by preload, afterload, and contractibility.

CO = HR X SV

The heart rate is controlled by the autonomic nervous system. Normally, if the heart rate decreases, stroke rate creases to compensate, but with cardiomyopathies, this may not occur, so bradycardia results in a sharp decline in cardiac output.

Administration of 12 lead ECG

The electrocardiogram provides a graphic representation of the electrical activity of the heart. It is indicated for chest pain, dyspnea, syncope, acute coronary syndrome, pulmonary embolism, and possible MI. The standard 12 lead ECG gives a picture of electrical activity from 12 perspectives through placement of 10 body leads:
- 4 limb leads are placed distally on the wrists and ankles (but may be placed more proximally if necessary),
- Precordial leads:
  - V1: right sternal border at 4th intercostal space
  - V2: left sternal border at 4th intercostal space
  - V3: Midway between V2 and V4
  - V4: Left midclavicular line at 5th intercostal space.
  - V5: Horizontal to V4 at left anterior axillary line.
  - V6: Horizontal to V5 at left midaxillary line.

In some cases, additional leads may be used:
- Right-sided leads are placed on the right in a mirror image of the left leads, usually to diagnose right ventricular infarction through ST elevation.

Hemodynamic monitoring and central venous/ right atrial pressure

Hemodynamic monitoring is the monitoring of blood flow pressures. In order for effective post-surgical cardiac functioning, the correct relationship between high and low pressures must be maintained. During surgery, catheters are placed; the most common sites are the left atrium, right atrium, and pulmonary artery or superior vena cava. Central venous pressure (CVP), the pressure in the right atrium or vena cava, is used to assess function of the right ventricles, preload, and flow of venous blood to the heart. Normal pressure ranges from 2-5 mm Hg but may be elevated after surgery to 6-8 mm Hg. Incorrect catheter placement or malfunctioning can affect readings.

- Increased CVP is related to overload of intravascular volume caused by decreased function, hypertrophy, or failure of the right ventricle; increased right ventricular afterload, tricuspid valve stenosis, regurgitation, or thrombus obstruction; or shunt from left ventricle to right atrium. It can also be caused by arrhythmias or cardiac tamponade.
- Decreased CVP is related to low intravascular volume, decreased preload, or vasodilation.

Non-invasive hemodynamic management

Thoracic electrical bioimpedance monitoring is a non-invasive method of monitoring hemodynamics (CO, blood flow, contractibility, pre- and after-load, pulmonary artery pressure). Electrodes placed on the thorax measure changes in electrical output associated with the volume of blood through the aorta and its velocity. The monitor to which the electrodes are attached converts the signals to waveforms. The heart rate is shown on an ECG monitor. The equipment calculates the cardiac output based on the heart rate and fluid volume. A typical bioimpedence monitor has 4 sets of bioimpedance electrodes and 3 ECG electrodes. Height, weight, and length of thorax are entered into the machine. Two sets of bioimpedance electrodes are placed at the base on the neck bilaterally and then two sets on each side of the chest. The distance between the neck electrodes and the chest electrodes (on the same side) must be entered into the machine. ECG leads are placed where they consistently monitor the QRS signal (they may need to be moved to achieve this).

Expanded jugular vein and mitral valve stenosis

Expanded jugular vein – This may be seen when the patient's head is raised to 45°. Make an approximation of the amount of tension there is on the venous area by getting the distance from the sternal angle to the uppermost place of venous pulsation. Jugular vein distension (JVD) is frequently seen in the elderly population. Pressure on this area is a sign of tension on the right heart chambers.

Mitral valve stenosis – Listen for a diastolic murmur. It will not be very loud. You may hear it on the apex of the heart.

Stress test – Also called an exercise tolerance test; the stress test is the most commonly used assessments to identify ischemic heart disease. It has a 98% precision rate for males older than 50 years of age who are identified with typical angina pectoris. It is not as precise if the patient has no indications of illness. This test may give a false-positive result if the patient is a male younger than 40 year of age with no symptoms, a premenopausal female who has no danger elements, or a patient taking digitalis.

Preventive measures recommended for patients at risk of developing renal calculi

There are many different types of renal calculi (kidney stones), and there are different risk factors and diseases associated with each. For the most part, however, diet modification is a good way to minimize the risk of kidney stone formation. Stones form in the kidney when certain minerals are present in high concentrations in the blood; dehydration contributes to the risk by further concentrating the minerals. Proper hydration is one of the best ways to prevent stone formation; drinking at least 2 liters of water a day will essentially "flush out" any debris that is present in the kidneys. Consuming foods that are low in sodium, nitrogen, and oxalate will reduce the risk of developing stones; patients who have suffered from stones in the past and are especially prone to them may also be placed on a low-protein diet. For patients with a predisposition to calcium stone formation, allopurinol may be an effective treatment as well.

Mechanical ventilation

Mechanical ventilation (MV) for status asthmaticus should be avoided if possible because of the danger of increased bronchospasm as well as barotrauma and decreased circulation. Aggressive medical management with β-adrenergic agonists, corticosteroids, and anticholinergics should be tried prior to ventilation. However, there are some absolute indications for the use of intubation and ventilation and a number of other indications that are evaluated on an individual basis.

Indications for MV	Relative indications for MV
<ul><li>Cardiac and/or pulmonary arrest.</li><li>Markedly depressed mental status (obtundation).</li><li>Severe hypoxia and/or apnea.</li><li>Bradycardia</li></ul>	<ul><li>Exhaustion/ muscle fatigue from exertion of trying to breathe.</li><li>Sharply diminished breath sounds and no audible wheezing.</li><li>Pulse paradoxus >20-40 mm Hg. If pulse paradoxus is absent, this is an indication of imminent respiratory arrest.</li><li>PaO_2 <70 mm Hg on 100% oxygen.</li><li>Deteriorating mental status.</li><li>Dysphonia.</li><li>Central cyanosis.</li><li>Increased hypercapnia.</li><li>Metabolic/respiratory acidosis</li></ul>

Tuberculosis

Tuberculosis - you will need to get a baseline liver function assessment before beginning any drugs for treatment. Check baseline color sight in a red/green assessment before using ethambutol. Check the ears before using streptomycin. Keep checking in with patients who have the condition in an active form. This condition must be reported to the state and regional health departments. If the patient was continually in contact with TB but had a negative skin test, the BCG vaccine may be needed. Once drug treatment has finished, check back in a year and keep checking for the condition's reappearance. Emphasize how vital it is to obey the rules of how to take the medication, even including Direct Observed Therapy (DOT) as a way to make sure the patient obeys. Emphasize the importance of balanced nutrition and instruct the patient on how to properly choose what he will eat.

Lumbar puncture

The lumbar puncture (spinal tap) is done between the 3rd and 4th or 4th and 5th lumbar vertebrae. The patient is in the lateral recumbent position with knees drawn toward the chest during the procedure. A local anesthetic is applied to prevent pain when the needle is inserted into the subarachnoid space to withdraw CSF and measure CSF pressure, which should be 70 to 200 mm H_2O.

Queckenstedt's test	CSF analysis
• Compress jugular veins on each side of *the neck during the* procedure. Note pressure and then release the veins and note pressure in 10-second intervals. Pressure should rise quickly with compression and fall quickly with release. Slower or no response indicates blockage of subarachnoid pathways.	• Normal values: • Clear and colorless. • Protein: 15-45 mg/dL. • Glucose: 60-80 mg/dL. • Lactic acid: <25.2 mg/dL • Culture: Negative • RBCs: 0 • WBCs: 0.5/mL

After a lumbar puncture, the patient should remain in the prone position for at least 3 hours to ensure that the needle puncture sites through the dural and arachnoid areas remain separate in order to reduce the chance of CSF leakage. If >20 mL of CSF is removed, then the patient should remain prone for 2 hours, side-lying (flat) for 2 or 3 hours and supine or prone for 6 additional hours. Relieving intracranial pressure by withdrawing CSF may cause herniation of the brain, so lumbar puncture should be done with care in the presence of increased ICP. The most common complaint is of spinal headache, which may occur within a few hours or several days of the procedure. Increased fluid intake may reduce risk of headache. If headache occurs, it may be treated with analgesics, fluids, and bed rest; however, if the headache is severe or persistent, an epidural blood patch may be done, with venous blood withdrawn and then injected into the epidural space at the site of the puncture to seal the leaking opening.

Status epilepticus

Status epilepticus is continuous seizure activity for greater than 30 minutes or repeated seizures that are not separated by a period of alertness. Status epilepticus is a life-threatening medical emergency. Establish an airway. Stabilize the patient's vital signs. Insert an IV and start benzodiazepines, phenytoin (Dilantin) or fosphenytoin. Midazolam is less likely to cause respiratory depression than lorazepam and diazepam. If you cannot find a good peripheral vein because of vessel constriction, use intraosseous (IO) access in the sternum. Use pentobarbital if other treatments fail. If your patient does not have a known history of epilepsy, find the underlying cause of the seizure. Order a CBC, metabolic profile, glucose, toxicology screen, and imaging. Anticipate fractures of the long bones and spinal damage. Complications of status epilepticus include: respiratory failure or aspiration; permanent brain damage; rhabdomyolysis; renal failure; hypoglycemia; hyperthermia; and death.

Cushing's syndrome

Cushing's syndrome (hypercortisolism) – The favored action is an operation. Take out adrenal tumors. Take out extra tissue growth. When a patient cannot have an operation, use radiation and medication. If the condition is caused by using steroids for a long time, stop using the medication slowly, lessen the amount of steroids used, and make a change in the medication routine so that it is only taken every other day.

Addison's disease (primary adrenocortical insufficiency) – Assessments include:
- Sodium amounts – Will be less than 130 mEq/L (regular is 135–145 mEq/L).
- Potassium level – Will be more than 5 mEq/L (regular is 3.5–5 mEq/L).
- BUN – Will be raised.
- Plasma renin – Will be raised.
- ACTH plasma – Will be raised.
- Serum sodium compared to potassium – > 30:1.
- Fasting blood glucose – Less than 50 mg/dL (regular is 60–115 mg/dL).
- Hematocrit – Will be raised.
- WBC – Will be less than normal.
- Eosinophils – More than usual.

Thoracic trauma

Fractured ribs are usually the result of severe trauma, such as blunt force from a motor vehicle accident or physical abuse. Underlying injuries should be expected according to the area of fractures:
- Upper 2 ribs: Injuries to trachea, bronchi, or great vessels.
- Right-sided ≥rib 8: Trauma to liver.
- Left-sided ≥ rib 8: Trauma to spleen.

Pain, often localized or experienced on respirations or compression of chest way may be the primary symptom of rib fractures, resulting in shallow breathing that can lead to atelectasis or pneumonia.

Treatment is primarily supportive as rib fractures usually heal in about 6 weeks: however, preventing pulmonary complications often necessitates adequate pain control. Underlying injuries are treated according to the type and degree of injury:
- Supplemental oxygen.
- Analgesia may include NSAIDs, intercostal nerve blocks, and narcotics.
- Pulmonary physiotherapy.

Agents used for pulmonary pharmacology

There are a wide range of agents used for pulmonary pharmacology, depending upon the type and degree of pulmonary disease. Agents include:
- Opioid analgesics: Use to provide both pain relief and sedation for those on mechanical ventilation to reduce sympathetic response. Medications may include fentanyl (Sublimaze®) or morphine sulfate (MS Contin®).

- Neuromuscular blockers: Used for induced paralysis of those who have not responded adequately to sedation, especially for intubation and mechanical ventilation. Medications may include pancuronium (Pavulon®) and vecuronium (Norcuron®). However, there is controversy about the use as induced paralysis has been linked to increased mortality rates, sensory hearing loss (pancuronium), atelectasis, and ventilation-perfusion mismatch.
- Human B-type natriuretic peptides: Used to reduce pulmonary capillary wedge pressure. Medications include nesiritide (Natrecor®).

Performing interventions for acute health problems

Acute health problems require interventions to provide essential care and treatment. Various conditions exist as older adults are at higher risk of developing certain illnesses and diseases. Older adults also need extra care and interventions because of physical changes to their bodies. For example, older adults can be more prone to skin tears because of impaired skin integrity. This also impacts the process of suturing, as it may be more difficult to suture and keep the sutures intact in an older person's skin. When administering a nerve block, the nurse should be aware of the patient's coagulation status as well as the potential for nerve damage from the procedure. With other types of interventions, the nurse must remain cognizant of the patient's physical status, knowing that changes in the older adult impact how well interventions are tolerated and that modifications may need to be made to account for aging.

Laboratory tests that should always be ordered on the febrile patient

When a patient has a fever, often the cause of the fever is not obvious. For this reason, laboratory tests, along with a thorough physical examination, can point the health care provider in the right direction. A white blood cell count should always be ordered. Although an elevated white cell count is not specific for infection, it is a positive indicator. Specifically, the presence of immature white cells in the blood (called a "left shift") is indicative of infection, because it means that white cells are being produced at an increased rate. A urinalysis should also be ordered to rule out a urinary tract infection as the cause of the fever, and a chest x-ray should be performed to rule out pneumonia. Blood cultures should also be ordered. If it is determined that the patient needs an antibiotic, a serum creatinine should be ordered to determine renal function because certain antibiotics should not be used in the setting of impaired renal function.

Vitamin D

Vitamin D is necessary for the intestinal absorption of both calcium and phosphorus, which is the reason that milk is fortified with vitamin D. It also aids in the reabsorption of calcium at the distal convoluted tubule in the kidney, and it promotes bone formation. Vitamin D is actually a prohormone called ergocalciferol, and requires ultraviolet light for synthesis into its active form, called cholecalciferol. Deficiency of vitamin D (whether due to lack of ingestion, lack of exposure to sunlight, or both) results in softening of the bones because of reabsorption of calcium and phosphorus, which form the mineral matrix of bone. In children, this bone softening is called rickets, and in adults it is called osteomalacia. Vitamin D deficiency may also contribute to osteoporosis. Symptoms of osteomalacia include bone pain (starting in the back and legs, then involving the chest and arms), muscle weakness, and fatigue. Nausea, vomiting, diarrhea, headache, and soft tissue calcification are all indicative of vitamin D toxicity.

Proteinuria

Proteinuria, or protein in the urine (over 150 mg per 24 hours), has a variety of benign, self-limiting causes, including intense exercise, acute illness, dehydration, and fever. Prolonged proteinuria is a result of 1 of 3 pathophysiologic mechanisms: glomerular, tubular, or overflow proteinuria. Glomerular disease, which is the most common cause of pathologic proteinuria, is the result of increased permeability of the glomerular capillaries. These capillaries are fenestrated, meaning that they are intentionally "leaky"; this allows for glomerular filtration. These fenestrations are small enough to restrict the passage of larger protein molecules into the urine; in the diseased glomerulus, however, these large proteins are leaked through into the urine. In patients with tubular disease, the proximal convoluted tubule does not reabsorb low molecular weight proteins from the glomerular filtrate, causing these proteins to be excreted into the urine. Overflow proteinuria is the result of overproduction of certain proteins; this occurs in diseases such as multiple myeloma and other gammopathies.

Glomerular filtration rate and creatinine clearance

Glomerular filtration rate (GFR) and creatinine clearance are used to evaluate the severity of chronic renal failure. The serum creatinine level can be used to estimate the GFR because decreased glomerular filtration will always result in an increase in the serum creatinine; this can be used as a quick determination of glomerular function. For a more accurate picture of glomerular function, however, the GFR must be calculated. For men, GFR is calculated by subtracting the patient's age from 140. This number is then multiplied by the patient's weight in kilograms. This number is then divided by the patient's serum creatinine times 72. For women, the same formula is used only the final number is multiplied by 0.85. Another equally accurate method of determining GFR is calculating the creatinine clearance. Creatinine clearance is equal to the patient's urine creatinine times the 24-hour urine volume divided by serum creatinine times 1,440.

Determining nutritional status

There are several markers of nutritional status. To determine the status of protein levels and consumption, the best markers are albumin, prealbumin, and transferrin. Albumin is the most abundant of all the serum proteins, and is important to the regulation of many of the body's physiologic functions; for this reason, it is often considered a "homeostasis" protein. Low levels of albumin (and prealbumin) can indicate poor nutrition. However, the levels of these proteins are also influenced by many other factors, including hydration, renal function, and liver function; the presence of a malignancy will also have an effect on serum protein levels. In the instance that other factors can be ruled out, low albumin (called hypoalbuminemia) is a fairly good indicator of poor nutritional status. Transferrin, another serum protein, is a good indicator of improving nutrition; transferrin levels rise fairly quickly when an individual begins to restore protein levels.

Diagnostic testing

First, it is important to remember that the positive and negative predictive values of a test are not absolute. For example, if you test a high-risk population for diabetes (say 180 out of 200 have the disease), and then you test a low-risk population (20 out of 200 have the disease), the sensitivity and specificity of the test will stay the same, but the predictive values will change. Also, a test that has less than 100% sensitivity and specificity is most useful for the patient with an equivocal or intermediate probability of disease, rather than a high-risk patient or a low-risk patient. One other important point to remember is that sensitivity and specificity are inversely related. If a diagnostic test is modified in order to increase its sensitivity, the specificity of the test will decrease, and vice versa.

Diagnostic and therapeutic uncertainty

Diagnosis and subsequent treatment are not easily arrived at for every patient because every patient is different. The clinical presentation of a heart attack, for example, may include severe chest pain, sweating, and nausea for one patient, and may have very mild, almost unnoticeable symptoms in another. Diagnostic uncertainty is especially prominent when dealing with diseases that have nonspecific symptoms; in these cases, it is important that the clinician recognize which of the possible diagnoses are life-threatening, and which are not. Ruling out the life-threatening possibilities should be higher on the clinician's list of priorities than the nonlife-threatening ones. Diagnostic testing, and subsequent treatment options, should also be evaluated according to the risks and benefits to the patient.

Clinical uncertainty

Although the degree of uncertainty is somewhat dependent on the patient, the clinical setting can have an influence on the degree of uncertainty that the clinician is likely to encounter. For example, a clinic, such as a dermatology clinic, is a setting in which the degree of uncertainty is likely to be low; this is because the clinic is nonemergent, and because the clinic treats a specific, limited group of diseases with which the clinicians are very familiar. An urgent care clinic would fall somewhere in the middle, because although there is a wider range of diagnostic possibility, life-threatening emergencies are rarely encountered. An emergency room or a trauma center, on the other hand, sees a high degree of uncertainty; the clinicians see a wide range of diagnostic possibilities, and are expected to work at a fast pace.

Evidence-based medicine

Evidence-based medicine (EBM) is defined as the "conscientious, explicit, and judicious use of current best evidence in making decisions about the care of individual patients." The goal of the practice of evidence-based medicine is to take information gained from scientific study and apply it to the practice of medicine. In other words, the direct outcome of the study is used to assess practicality and efficacy in clinical practice. The goal of the studies behind EBM is to determine and identify all the risks associated with a particular treatment, as well as all the benefits. Once the risks and the benefits have been identified, they can be weighed against one another to determine the overall risk/benefit ratio for that particular treatment plan.

Evidence-based guidelines

Steps to evidence-based practice guidelines include:
- Focus on the topic/methodology: This includes outlining possible interventions/treatments for review, choosing patient populations and settings and determining significant outcomes. Search boundaries (such as types of journals, types of studies, dates of studies) should be determined.
- Evidence review: This includes review of literature, critical analysis of studies, and summarizing of results, including pooled meta-analysis.
- Expert judgment: Recommendations based on personal experience from a number of experts may be utilized, especially if there is inadequate evidence based on review, but this subjective evidence should be explicated acknowledged.
- Policy considerations: This includes cost-effectiveness, access to care, insurance coverage, availability of qualified staff, and legal implications.
- Policy: A written policy must be completed with recommendations. Common practice is to utilize letter guidelines, with "A" the most highly recommended, usually based the quality of supporting evidence.
- Review: The completed policy should be submitted to peers for review and comments before instituting the policy.

Evidenced based clinical guidelines

Evidence based clinical guidelines are recommendations for clinical care practices. These guidelines are supported by evidence based practice measures, meaning that the evidence to support the guidelines has been reviewed through a systematic process. Evidence based practice uses the latest clinical research results and practices to define the best methods. It is this evidence that is used to develop the guidelines. Once developed, clinicians should use these guidelines to direct their practices. Evidence based guidelines may also be used for other measures, such as educational tools for patients and their families. They may back up the practice of clinicians so that if a measure is put into question, such as by insurance companies, the guidelines can be used as a standard of measurement. Evidence based clinical practice guidelines are also useful for quality improvement measures, to determine where upgrades can be made.

Standard of care

The standard of care is the criteria or guideline provided to nurses and health care providers that defines the quality of care that should be given. High-quality care should be given everywhere, but the standard of care can vary between specific types of care areas, and the related tasks and decisions depend on the area. For example, tasks associated with standards of care for cardiac patients in a critical care unit will vary from task standards for residents of long-term care facilities. Although the standards will be high in quality in both areas, the tasks associated with each are different. Standards of care can be broken down into several steps, including assessment of the patient, nursing diagnosis, identifying patient outcomes, planning for nursing interventions, implementing the interventions, and finally, evaluating the results. Following these steps through the nursing process will help to fully implement the standard of care.

Common standards of care and clinical guidelines

Standards of care and clinical guidelines vary between populations and levels of acuity of care provided. Common standards of care and clinical guidelines among older adults include such measures as patient safety, pharmacologic intervention, and quality of life. Older adults may be at higher risk of falls, impaired skin integrity, the development of certain illnesses or disabilities, and impaired mobility. Common clinical guidelines for nurses working with this population center on improving patient safety and mobility to avoid the risk of falls, improving nutrition to avoid malnutrition and maintain skin integrity, and assist with health screenings and medication administration. Older adults may take many different types of medications to manage their health conditions. Clinical guidelines are in place to assist patients with medication administration as well as knowledge of side effects. Additionally, common clinical guidelines and care standards exist that can help to maintain quality of life among older adults, such as addressing depression and mental health issues.

Subjective Global Assessment and Prognostic Nutritional Index

Assessing the nutritional status of the hospital inpatient is an important part of forming a care plan. The 2 screening tools that are most commonly used are the Subjective Global Assessment (SGA) and the Prognostic Nutritional Index (PNI). The SGA provides a nutritional assessment based on both the patient history and current symptoms. The patient is asked about any changes in weight, and is also asked questions about his or her diet. The presence of symptoms that may lead to weight loss and poor nutritional status, such as diarrhea, nausea, and vomiting, as well as water retention (edema) and muscle wasting (cachexia), is also included in the SGA. The PNI is also used as an indicator of malnutrition, and is especially helpful in determining how well a patient will recover from surgery; the PNI assesses nutritional status through the measurement of serum proteins such as albumin and transferrin, combined with a skinfold measurement and a cutaneous hypersensitivity test (as an indicator of immune function).

Stressed starvation and simple starvation

When the body is stressed, the physiological changes that result from starvation are altered because of the response of stress hormones such as cortisol, as well as epinephrine and norepinephrine. Cortisol, a hormone released during stress, causes blood glucose levels to remain elevated through increased gluconeogenesis (breakdown of proteins to form glucose). The persistent high level of glucose leads to insulin resistance, which further perpetuates the high blood glucose level. In addition, the stimulation of gluconeogenesis by cortisol results in a depletion of protein, which is why stressed starvation may also be referred to as hypoalbuminemic malnutrition. Because gluconeogenesis is continuous, fat stores are not used up as they are during simple starvation; this leads to a wasting of muscle mass without loss of fat stores, so that the individual may still be perceived as "obese" although he or she is not receiving enough nutrition.

Body fat distribution

Another example of an anthropometric measurement is the waist to hip ratio; to calculate this ratio, the individual divides the circumference of his or her waist (measured at the level of the umbilicus) by the circumference or his or her hips (measured where the buttocks are

- 95 -

at their widest point). This helps to determine the distribution of an individual's body fat, which is an important indicator of health. An individual who tends to store fat around the abdomen, arms, and back ("apple-shaped" body type), for example, is at a greater risk of cardiovascular disease and diabetes than is an individual who accumulates fat in the thighs and buttocks ("pear-shaped" body type). It has been shown that individuals with excess abdominal (visceral) fat usually accumulate fat in that area because of a growing insulin resistance, which can lead to diabetes and cardiovascular problems. For women, the ideal waist to hip ratio is less than 0.8, and for men less than 1.0.

Anthropometry

Anthropometry is defined as the measurement of either a part of the body or the entire body; basic examples include height and weight measurements. Weight is an important measurement when determining the caloric requirements of an individual; the ideal weight is usually determined based on the individual's height. Of course, no two people are alike, and the ideal weight for one may not be the ideal weight for another. Perhaps the most accurate method to date for calculating ideal body weight is the body mass index (BMI). BMI is typically calculated by dividing the weight (in kilograms) by the square of the height (in meters). A BMI greater than 25 is typically considered to be overweight, while a BMI greater than 30 is considered obese. The Hamwi equation provides a rough estimate of ideal weight; a 5 ft woman is considered to be 100 lbs; for each inch over 5 ft, 5 pounds are added, so that a woman measuring 5'7" has an ideal weight of 135 lbs.

Obesity

Obesity is usually defined based on either BMI or ideal body weight as calculated using the Hamwi equation. Using BMI as a reference, obesity is defined as a BMI greater than 27, while a BMI greater than 30 is considered severely (or morbidly) obese. Using an ideal body weight calculation, weight greater than 20% above the ideal body weight is considered obese, while weight greater than 40% above the ideal body weight is considered to be severely obese. Although these are good guidelines to use when evaluating an overweight individual, other factors must be considered. Factors that have been shown to correlate to obesity include lack of physical activity, poor or inappropriate diet, genetics, and economic class.

Parenteral nutrition

Although parenteral nutrition is a great method for providing nutrition to severely ill patients who cannot tolerate enteral support, it should be avoided unless absolutely necessary because there are many risk factors associated with this type of nutritional support. Most of the problems that occur during treatment with parenteral nutrition are related to the indwelling catheter; it is a common site for infection, and, in the compromised patient, sepsis is both more likely and more dangerous. Catheters may also move or dislodge, causing discomfort and other problems; they can become clogged, and clots can form and then break off, resulting in thrombosis. Air bubbles in the tubing can enter the bloodstream, causing an air embolus. The patient may also have problems tolerating the nutritional supplements, and it can be difficult to control glucose levels as well.

Enteral support and parenteral support

Enteral nutrition is a method of providing nutrition to a patient through a tube; the tube may be placed in either the nose (a nasogastric tube), the stomach (a percutaneous endoscopic gastrostomy [PEG] tube), or the small bowel (a percutaneous endoscopic jejunal [J] tube). When the tube has been placed, nutrition can be administered through the tube and absorbed by the patient's digestive system. Various enteric formulas exist, and the choice is dependent on the nutritional requirements of the patient. Parenteral nutrition (also called total parenteral nutrition [TPN]) is a method of providing nutrition that completely bypasses the digestive system by administering nutrition through an intravenous line. Enteral support is the preferred method of providing nutrition, although in patients suffering from some compromise of the gastrointestinal tract, parenteral nutrition is the only option.

Determining the caloric requirements of critically ill patients

When an individual requires hospitalization for a critical illness, his or her caloric requirements must be determined so that normal body function is maintained, and so that recovery is as quick as possible. There are many factors that must be considered when attempting to determine the requirements of an ill patient. First, the age of the patient is important. If the patient is a growing child or adolescent, he or she will have very different nutritional requirements than an elderly individual would have. Also to be considered is the physical and nutritional status of the patient, independent of the illness. A patient who is normally very active would have different requirements than an overweight, sedentary individual. Along the same lines, comorbidities, such as diabetes and atherosclerosis, need to be considered, as well as overall stress levels of the patient.

Harris Benedict equation

The Harris Benedict equation is a useful tool when determining the caloric requirements necessary for the critically ill patient. The goal of the equation is to determine the resting energy expenditure of the patient; that is, what is the baseline energy level that is required to maintain physiological function. The equation considers the factors of age, weight, and height when calculating caloric requirements. For women, the resting energy expenditure is calculated as $655 + (9.6 \times \text{weight in kilograms}) + (1.7 \times \text{height in centimeters}) - (4.7 \times \text{age in years})$. For men, resting energy expenditure is calculated as $66 + (13.7 \times \text{weight in kilograms}) + (5 \times \text{height in centimeters}) - (6.8 \times \text{age in years})$. Additional modifications can be made to the equation to accommodate differences in activity and stress levels.

Occupational therapy

The philosophy of occupational therapy is based on the idea that occupation (meaning, loosely, either an activity or activities in which an individual engages) is a basic human need, one that is important to an individual's health and overall well-being in that it is in and of itself therapeutic in nature. The basic assumptions of occupational therapy are based on the idea of occupational therapy as stated by its creator, William Rush Dunton. Dunton states that occupational therapy is a human need because an individual's occupation has an effect on his or her health and general well-being. It creates structure in the individual's life, and allows for him or her to manage and organize time. Another assumption is that individuals have different sets of values, and therefore will value different occupations; for each person, however, the occupation that he or she chooses is meaningful to him or her.

Occupational therapy is defined as the use of creative activities in the treatment of disabled individuals, whether they are disabled physically or mentally. The purpose of occupational therapy is to provide disabled individuals with the skills that are necessary to live life as fully and independently as possible; after completion of occupational therapy, the individual should be able to perform at his or her maximum potential. The occupational therapist will typically provide the patient with interventions tailored to his or her disability. The OT will also visit the patient's home and/or place of employment in order to assess potential problems and provide adaptive solutions. As part of occupational therapy, the patient will receive regular assessments of his or her skills, as well as specific training. The occupational therapist is also responsible for educating the patient's family, caretakers, friends, and coworkers.

Although occupational therapy is an important part of the overall rehabilitation process for hospitalized individuals, it is also beneficial in other areas, because occupational therapy deals not only with physical disabilities, but with emotional and cognitive disabilities as well. Occupational therapy as related to physical disabilities may be practiced in outpatient clinics, pediatric hospitals or units, acute care rehabilitation facilities, and long-term, or comprehensive, inpatient rehabilitation centers. Occupational therapy as related to mental disabilities may be practiced in mental health clinics, acute and long-term psychiatric hospitals, prisons, and gateway or halfway houses. Occupational therapists may also work at schools, childcare facilities, workplaces, or shelters, or they may even work with individuals in their own homes.

Assessing potential for rehabilitation

There are various factors that are considered when assessing a patient to determine whether he or she will benefit from rehabilitation. A patient with the inability to perform any of the ADLs will automatically be considered for rehabilitation; at this point, however, other factors must be considered. First and foremost is whether or not the patient has a desire to improve his or her functions through rehabilitation; if the patient is not interested in improvement, the rehabilitation potential is poor. If the patient wants to improve function and increase independence, the potential for rehabilitation is greater. Another factor is whether or not the patient has support at home; even if the patient improves greatly during his or her rehabilitation stay, he or she will still most likely need some support at home. If the patient has no support at home, rehabilitation may eventually fail.

Rehabilitation

Rehabilitation is an area of health care that is dedicated to helping patients improve and/or restore functions and abilities after a disease or injury. Although rehabilitation is usually thought of in relation to physical therapy (which is one of the many areas of rehabilitation), it also encompasses drug and alcohol rehabilitation, as well as occupational therapy for physically and mentally ill patients. The general goals of all types of rehabilitation include an improvement in overall function; the promotion of independence, satisfaction, and well-being; and the preservation of the individual's self esteem in the face of illness or debilitating disease or injury.

When a patient is to be considered for rehabilitation, he or she must undergo a rather extensive evaluation in order to increase the likelihood that he or she will succeed during rehabilitation. This process of evaluation, which includes various interventions, should take place in the early stages of illness, when the patient is still in the hospital. The goal is to forestall any secondary complications that may inhibit the rehabilitation process. These interventions include health management, in which the patient and family are educated about his or her disease(s); nutritional status assessment and support; initiation of bowel and bladder management in order to prevent infection; exercises; assessment of cognitive function; and education involving self-esteem, relationship roles, sexual activity, and coping mechanisms.

There are some diseases, illnesses, and injuries that almost always require rehabilitation at some point during their course; in these cases, rehabilitation may be initiated before the patient even leaves the hospital to be transferred to a rehabilitation facility. It is important to know which diseases usually require rehabilitation, because the sooner evaluation and rehabilitation are initiated, the better the patient's chance of recovery. The following are diseases, illnesses, and injuries that commonly require rehabilitation: AIDS, amyotrophic lateral sclerosis (ALS), limb amputation, traumatic or ischemic brain injury, spinal cord injury, burns, Guillain-Barré syndrome, hip or knee replacement, multiple sclerosis (MS), and most types of cancer.

There are various kinds of rehabilitation settings, depending on the needs of the patient. Once the need for rehabilitation has been determined, and the patient has been evaluated regarding specific rehabilitation needs, he or she can be placed in an appropriate rehabilitation setting. A long-term acute care hospital is a rehabilitation facility that is best for patients who are physically and psychologically stable, but are receiving medical treatment such as dialysis or ventilation, and thus require medical support. A subacute care unit is appropriate for patients who require more limited treatment, such as cancer patients. A comprehensive inpatient rehabilitation facility is just what the name suggests; it addresses the needs of a broad range of different patients, from burn victims to amputees. The comprehensive rehabilitation center has a "team" of medical specialists that includes a rehabilitation medicine physician, nurses trained in rehabilitation, occupational therapists, physical therapists, social workers, and speech-language pathologists. Outpatient rehab is designed for the high-functioning patient who can return home after rehab sessions.

Pain management

Promoting a caring and supportive environment means ensuring that the patient is comfortable. According to Joint Commission guidelines and Federal law, all patients have to right to pain management, and this applies to all ages. It's not enough to recognize this; procedures must be in place to assure that all staff are committed to reducing pain and that patients/families be apprised of the right and benefits of pain management. There are steps that the institution can take in this process:
- Create an interdisciplinary team to research, provide guidelines, and communicate goals.
- Assess pain management procedures already in place to determine effectiveness or need for change.
- Establish a minimum standard that should be legally followed.
- Clarify responsibility for pain control and imbed this in the standards of practice.
- Provide information about pain control to all levels of care providers.

- Educate patients to understand they are entitled to rapid response.
- Educate staff to institutionalize pain management.

All patients have the right to appropriate assessment and management of pain. Caregivers should encourage all patients to report their pain and follow through with pain-relieving treatments. Assessments for pain must be appropriate for the individual patient and address all aspects of their pain. Both the patient and family should be included in the assessment process. The most accurate indicator of pain is the patient's own description. It is always subjective: The clinician should accept and respect the patient's report of pain. Each person's pain experience is unique and dependent on many contributing factors such as heredity, energy level, coping skills, and prior experiences. Physiological and behavioral observations should not replace information obtained directly from the patient when it can be communicated. Pain can be present without physiological evidence or cause; pain in such cases should not be immediately assigned to psychological causes. Chronic pain can create an overall lower threshold of tolerance for pain and other stimuli. Unrelieved pain has adverse effects on all aspects of the patient's life.

Low back pain

Low back pain (LBP) – To alleviate hurting, use salicylates or acetaminophen, nonsteroidal anti-inflammatory drugs (NSAIDs), and opiates in some circumstances. Medicine used to loosen up the muscles may be used temporarily (1–2 weeks), but stay away from these if the patient is older. For radiculopathy, the initial medication is 5-day steroid dose pack. Make an appointment for another check-up a week later. When the patient has not gotten better in that week, he should see an expert to get an epidural steroid injection (ESI). Traction is another alternative. Use back and abdominal physical activity to keep it from happening or coming back. Do not do these exercises when an attack is occurring. Walking is more useful for this condition than running. Back rubs can help. Sometimes the patient has a psychosocial issue that adds to the problem, such as anxiety, depression, family aggression, no coping mechanisms, or marriage and family issues. The patient can go back to his or her job as long as action is restricted. They must learn to handle stress.

Falls

Falls are extremely common in the elderly population and are a significant cause of physical and psychological injury. Risk factors for falls include age over 75, living alone, history of a previous fall, need for a cane or walker, and cognitive, visual or neurological impairment. Elderly patients should be questioned about falls at each visit. An important part of the history is an assessment of the living situation and potential hazards that may exist there. Patients should also be questioned about medications they are taking. Medications that can increase a patient's risk for falling include any drug that is sedating, cardiac and antihypertensive medications, and hypoglycemic drugs. A patient with a history of falling should have a detailed physical exam. Special attention should be given to orthostatic vital signs, joints, and neurological exam, including visual, hearing and nutritional status. The goals of intervention are aimed at reducing the risk of falling. Interventions include education, minimizing risk factors, correcting any underlying cause, and reducing hazards in the home.

Colorectal cancer

Colorectal cancer – The patient will need any tumors removed with an operation or a resection, the choice of which is contingent upon how deep is the cancer is. If it has spread when the problem is identified, there is a more negative prediction for the future, and palliative medical attention will be needed. If the patient needs resection, there is commonly a need for temporary colostomy. Watch the patient for indications of not enough body fluid while getting colon preps.

The American Cancer Society advises colon cancer screens for patients with an average chance of getting it, starting when the patient turns 50. This includes assessments for fecal occult blood every year, flexible sigmoidoscopy done in 5-year increments, double-contrast barium enema done in 5-year increments, and colonoscopy done in 10-year increments.

Esophageal cancer

Esophageal cancer is most typically seen in men older than 50. Miners, construction workers, and dry cleaners tend to develop it through occupational exposure to silica dust and solvents. African-Americans are prone to squamous carcinoma. Caucasians are prone to adenocarcinoma. Risk factors for developing esophageal cancer include: Excessive alcohol use; tobacco use; obesity (BMI >25); diet lacking in Vitamin A, B_1, C and selenium; drinking hot liquids; radiotherapy; and Barrett's esophagus (erosion due to GERD). Esophageal cancer is sometimes associated with achalasia, esophageal webs or tylosis. Patients usually present with: Difficulty swallowing; pain between the shoulder blades; a sensation of food sticking in the throat or chest; unintentional weight loss; voice hoarseness; hiccups; and vomiting blood. Confirm your diagnosis with upper endoscopy and biopsy. Early-stage cancer can be treated surgically and is sometimes curative. Late-stage esophageal cancer cannot be treated surgically. Chemotherapy and radiation are palliative in advanced cases.

Ovarian cancer

Although there are no direct causes that have been definitively linked to ovarian cancer, there are multiple factors that are attributed to the risk of developing the disease. Perhaps the strongest indicator that a woman may develop ovarian cancer is a genetic mutation of either the BRCA1 or BRCA2 gene, which also carries an increased risk of developing breast cancer. Increased age is associated with an increased risk of ovarian cancer, as is young age at menarche, and nulliparity. Conversely, multiparity and the use of oral contraceptives are linked to a reduced risk of developing ovarian cancer. Although ovarian cancer is notorious for its lack of symptoms (and thus its advanced stage at diagnosis), there are a few (however general) symptoms that are associated with ovarian cancer, including pelvic pain, bloating, urinary urgency, and feeling full very quickly when eating.

Hospice care

The name hospice is derived from the word hospitality. Hospice care is based on the philosophy of the acceptance of the death. The goal of hospice care is to provide a pain-free, dignified setting in which patients can spend their final days. Hospice care is generally recommended when a patient has less than six months to live and conventional treatments have either been exhausted or are considered inappropriate. Hospice care is available in many different settings, including the home, hospital and extended care facilities. Hospice care is generally accomplished by a multidisciplinary team including physicians, nurses, therapists, social workers and clergy. Regular meetings with the team and the family are critical to the success of hospice care.

Red eye

Causes: Foreign body; chemical burn; conjunctivitis; corneal abrasion; blepharitis; preseptal and orbital cellulitis; and improper contact lens use.

First Aid: If patient has chemical burns, or an unembedded foreign body, flush eyes with sterile saline.

Diagnosis: Take a detailed history. Carefully examine eyelid, orbit, pupil, and extraocular muscles. Test visual acuity. Visualize fundi with ophthalmoscope. Apply fluorescein stain. Use a slit lamp to see abrasions. Measure intraocular pressure with tonometer; normal range is 10 to 20 mm/Hg.

Treatment: Instill 2 drops of tetracaine 0.5% to relieve pain. Prevent secondary infection by placing a large dab of sulfacetamide 10% eye ointment in the lower conjunctival sac. Use double sterile patch for corneal ulceration. Reassess patient after 24 hours.

Refer to ophthalmologist within 24 hours if: Decreased visual acuity; abnormal pupils; penetrated cornea; large or central ulcer; severe pain; rust ring indicates an embedded metallic foreign body (e.g., iron filings); pressure exceeds 21 mm/Hg.

Refer to ophthalmologist within 48 to 72 hours if: Abrasion does not respond to treatment after 48 hours.

Patient rights to keep in mind when planning care

The rights of patients must be a top priority when planning patient care and obtaining care from outside providers. The patient has a right to make any decisions they are capable of making regarding their care. The practitioner, the health care team, and sometimes the courts have a say in how capable the patient is of making decisions for himself, and the case manager helps with this evaluation. This is done by determining the patient's functional status, which includes their mental and emotional status. If the patient is competent, their requests regarding where and when care is provided should be honored whenever possible. If the level of care cannot be provided where the patient requests it, the reason the service or provider is not being used must be documented in the medical record.

Transitional care planning and discharge care planning

Transitional care planning is a general term which describes any focused planning for a patient moving through the health care system. It is an all-encompassing term which describes the entire care process, from admission to discharge. There are laws regarding transitional planning that are enforced by legislation. They guide the case manager, and have written performance standards which allow the case manager to meet accreditation standards in the form of policies and procedures. Discharge planning is also mandated by federal law, and is part of transitional care planning. Transitional care planning includes working with other providers and professionals to meet the patient's needs and negotiate with the payer for reimbursement

The transitional process is part of the case management process, and involves assessing everything possible about the patient, including his or her condition, his or her family, and everything else that relates to the disease and the current admission. The process starts with admission to the hospital or the episode of care. The case manager assesses and identifies actual or potential problems, and involves all interdisciplinary team members in the coordination of activities and treatment plans. This includes brokerage of services or referrals to other providers. The interdisciplinary team involves family members or other support people, and prepares plans for education and training to meet the needs of the patient. The goal is to plan and provide the best care possible at the best price for the patient.

Discharge planning begins as soon as a patient is admitted to hospital. The health care team starts educating the patient right away about what to expect and what milestones need to be met before discharge. They also interview the patient about what they want to see happen upon discharge. A patient may have had many admissions, and will know from the beginning that they can no longer handle self care at home. The interdisciplinary team would take this information into account when developing a plan of care for this hospitalization and start making contacts with facilities that may be able to handle the patient upon discharge. Discharge planning must be started early to shorten the length of the hospital stay and plan appropriate post-hospital care. These issues are interconnected, everyone should help with the coordination of and communication between all providers and payers.

Discharge planning is a formal process that allows care providers to coordinate the individual needs of the patient extending beyond their time in a hospital or long-term-care setting. This assessment process examines how to provide the appropriate provider care once they no longer meet criteria for hospitalization. Also considered is an understanding of the patient's insurance and benefit coverage to ensure that needed services will be available without unreasonable financial burden. The patient must receive clear and accurate teaching about their condition and self-care as well as community resources that will be available to them.

Neuman's framework

The development of the Neuman's framework was meant to provide nursing caregivers with a guideline to help them understand the role he or she has in promoting health and well-being among individual patients and communities alike. Because each patient has individual stressors that are unique to him or her, it is necessary for the APRN to identify these stressors and tailor his or her approach to the patient (or family, or community). By identifying these unique stressors, the APRN can assess the patient's risk regarding certain diseases and illnesses. Risk factor analysis and assessment is a necessary step toward educating the patient. Once the APRN identifies these risk factors, he or she can discuss these with the patient and offer suggestions for risk reduction, starting the patient on the road to a healthier life.

The Neuman framework of nursing health promotion is a broad, flexible perspective that can be applied to nearly any situation that the acute care nurse may encounter in practice.

The framework is based around the idea of a "client system," which may represent an individual patient, or it may represent a family, group, or entire community. In the Neuman framework, the client system is an ever-changing, open network that is constantly interacting with both the internal environment and the external environment. The role of the APRN in this framework is to identify stressors within these environments that are harming or have the potential to harm the client system. Once the APRN has identified these stressors, it is his or her job to educate the client system about them, and to help them work through them, so that the client system can maintain a healthy, balanced environment.

Substance abuse

Many people with substance abuse (alcohol or drugs) are reluctant to disclose this information, but there are a number of indicators that are suggestive of substance abuse:

Physical signs	Other signs
<ul><li>Needle tracks on arms or legs.</li><li>Burns on fingers or lips.</li><li>Pupils abnormally dilated or constricted, eyes watery.</li><li>Slurring of speech, slow speech.</li><li>Lack of coordination, instability of gait.</li><li>Tremors.</li><li>Sniffing repeatedly, nasal irritation.</li><li>Persistent cough.</li><li>Weight loss.</li><li>Dysrhythmias.</li><li>Pallor, puffiness of face.</li></ul>	<ul><li>Odor of alcohol/marijuana on clothing or breath.</li><li>Labile emotions, including mood swings, agitation, and anger.</li><li>Inappropriate, impulsive, and/or risky behavior.</li><li>Lying.</li><li>Missing appointments.</li><li>Difficulty concentrating/short term memory loss, disoriented/confused.</li><li>Blackouts.</li><li>Insomnia or excessive sleeping.</li><li>Lack of personal hygiene.</li></ul>

Drug screening

A drug screen is used to determine use of illicit drugs. Testing varies according to the type of drug used, duration of use, and time of use. Different types of screens include:
- Serum: Most drugs can be detected within 24 hours and for up to 3-5 days, but this varies.
- Saliva: Similar to serum, drugs can usually be detected within 1 to 3 hours of use and for 2 or 3 days afterward.
- Perspiration: The person wears a special patch for up to 2 weeks to evaluate chronic drug use.
- Urine: Drugs show up in the urine in about 6 to 8 hours, but tests can be inaccurate if people dilute urine by drinking 1 to 2 liters of fluids or add adulterants that change the chemical makeup of the urine.
- Hair: Drugs and alcohol can usually be detected in hair within about two weeks of use and remain for about 90 days.

Decision making

The number of tasks assigned to an APRN can have an adverse effect both on the APRN's decision-making abilities and on the safety of the patient. If the APRN has too many things to do in too short a time, he or she will not be able to dedicate the time necessary for diagnosis, decision-making, and treatment, and the patient will suffer. If the APRN is missing information that is essential to diagnosis, such as a complete history, or a list of current medications, he or she cannot make well-informed decisions that would be best for the patient. Behaviors not encouraging of productive thought include daydreaming, multitasking, and other distractions that make it impossible for the APRN to dedicate his or her full attention to the clinical decision-making process.

Progression of risk assessment

It is important for the primary care nurse practitioner (PCNP) and the acute care nurse practitioner (ACNP) to communicate with one another concerning risk assessment. The relationship becomes clear as you consider the role of each caregiver. Assume that patient X presents to his PCNP complaining of shortness of breath. The PCNP, through the history and physical examination, can narrow the differential diagnosis to a cardiac cause, and then refer the patient to cardiology. The ACNP, in reviewing the information from the PCNP, can then begin screening tests (if they have not already been done). With all of this information together (the history and physical, the risk assessment provided by the PCNP, and the test results), the ACNP can develop a treatment plan for the patient.

Primary, secondary, and tertiary prevention

Risk assessment can be divided into 3 different prevention strategies; for the APRN, this depends largely on the point at which he or she intervenes with the patient. APRNs that work in community health clinics, public health, urgent care, and primary care, for example, will most often be focused on primary and secondary prevention; the acute care nurse practitioner, on the other hand, is typically concerned with secondary and tertiary prevention. Primary prevention involves patient education concerning stressors, allowing the patient to identify and defend against them; the focus in this case is on illness prevention. If an illness is identified, secondary prevention focuses on immediate treatment and alleviation of symptoms. Tertiary prevention focuses on the reduction of future stressors, as well as preparation of the patient to readapt to the environment.

Risk assessment and illness prevention

The US Department of Health and Human Services' Guide to Clinical Preventive Services states that there are 2 important factors that must be considered above all else when evaluating a patient for preventive services. First, the APRN must consider how effective a clinical intervention will be in improving the outcome of the patient, and, second, the APRN must consider what the overall leading causes of mortality and morbidity are. The leading causes of mortality and morbidity can be assessed by population, whether it is age, sex, or some other risk-associated population. Once the patient has been assessed for the appropriate population-related risk factors, and once the APRN has determined the best intervention based on these risk factors, preventive services can be initiated.

Collecting data for use in risk assessment

The APRN must determine a patient's risk for developing diseases or illnesses based on a multitude of factors; again, Neuman framework outlines those areas that the APRN should consider and investigate when assessing a patient's risk. The first step in any patient interview process, of course, is the detailed patient history. The information that the patient history provides for the APRN is indispensable; therefore, the APRN should attempt to elicit as much information as possible during the history-taking process, including information about the patient's family life, social life, and psychological well-being. In addition to the comprehensive history, the APRN should also expect to gain information about risk factors from the physical examination of the patient. Once the APRN has developed a risk profile for the patient based on this information, he or she can proceed to the next step in the prevention process.

Determining risk

Typically, when trying to identify the amount of risk, the first step is hazard identification. Essentially what this means is that the adversity of the outcome (whether the risk is associated with chemical exposure, alcohol consumption, cigarette smoking, or any other risky behavior or situation) is determined based on supportive information; for example, the lifetime risk of developing emphysema in individuals with a 40 pack-year smoking history. The next step is the "dose-response analysis," the aim of which is to determine the correlation between the amount of exposure and the degree of adversity. Exposure assessment and quantification, the third step, aims to determine the probable amount of exposure that each individual within the population will receive.

Behavior modification and compliance rate

Education, like all interventions, must be evaluated for effectiveness. Two determinants of effectiveness include:
- Behavior modification involves thorough observation and measurement, identifying behavior that needs to be changed and then planning and instituting interventions to modify that behavior. An ACNP can use a variety of techniques, including demonstrations of appropriate behavior, reinforcement, and monitoring until new behavior is adopted consistently. This is especially important when longstanding procedures and habits of behavior are changed.
- Compliance rates are often determined by observation, which should be done at intervals and on multiple occasions, but with patients, this may depend on self-reports. Outcomes is another measure of compliance; that is, if education is intended to improve patient health and reduce risk factors and that occurs, it is a good indication that there is compliance. Compliance rates are calculated by determining the number of events/procedures and degree of compliance.

Outcomes evaluation and evidence-based practice

Outcomes evaluation is an important component of evidence-based practice, which involves both internal and external research. All treatments are subjected to review to determine if they produce positive outcomes, and policies and protocols for outcomes evaluation should be in place. Outcomes evaluation includes the following:

- Monitoring over the course of treatment involves careful observation and record keeping that notes progress, with supporting laboratory and radiographic evidence as indicated by condition and treatment.
- Evaluating results includes reviewing records as well as current research to determine if outcomes are within acceptable parameters.
- Sustaining involves continuing treatment, but continuing to monitor and evaluate.
- Improving means to continue the treatment but with additions or modifications in order to improve outcomes.
- Replacing the treatment with a different treatment must be done if outcomes evaluation indicates that current treatment is ineffective.

Incorporating patient/family rights into plan of care

In order for patient/family rights to be incorporated into the plan of care, the care plan needs to be designed as a collaborative effort that encourages participation of patients and family members. There are a number of different programs that can be useful, such as including patients and families on advisory committees. Additionally, assessment tools, such as surveys for patients/families, can be utilized to gain insight in the issues that are important to them. While infants and small children and sometimes the elderly cannot speak for themselves, "patient" is generally understood to include not only the immediate family but also other groups or communities who have an interest in the care of an individual or individuals. Because many hospital stays are now short-term, programs that include follow-up interviews and assessments are especially valuable in determining if the needs of the patient/family were addressed in the care plan.

Healthcare Systems

Delivery of care

The delivery of care is impacted by a numerous forces:
- Social forces are increasing demand for access to treatment and medical services, both traditional and complementary. As society views equitable medical care as a right, then delivery of care must be available to all.
- Political forces affect medical care as the Federal and state governments increasingly become purchasers of medical care, imposing their guidelines and limitations on the medical system.
- Regulatory forces may be local, state, or Federal and can have a profound effect of delivery of care and services, differing from one state or region to another.
- Economic forces, such as managed care or cost-containment committees, try to contain costs to insurers and facilities by controlling access to and duration of treatment, and limiting products. Economic pressure is working to prevent duplication of services in a geographical area, and providers are creating networks to purchase supplies and equipment directly.

Disaster

A disaster is an event where many people are exposed to hazards that results in injury, death, and damage to property. There are a number of hazards that have the potential to lead to a disaster situation. In general, they can be classified as natural, technological, or caused by human conflict. Some specific examples of each are as follows:
- NATURAL: Firestorms, flood, land shift, tornado, epidemic, earthquake, volcano, hurricane, high winds, blizzard, heat wave.
- TECHNOLOGICAL: Hazmat spills, explosions, utility failure, building collapse, transportation accident, power outage, nuclear accident, dam failure, fire, water loss, ruptured gas main.
- HUMAN CONFLICT: Riots, strikes, suicide bombings, bomb threat, employee violence, mass shootings, equipment sabotage, hostage events, transportation disruption, weapons of mass destruction, computer viruses/worms.

Disaster management plan

There are many different types of disaster management plans. Regardless of the type, however, there are several basic steps for its development. To begin with, a planning team must be established that includes representatives from all levels within the organization. The planning team is responsible for putting together a timeline for completion of the plan as well as an estimation of the costs, fees, and resources necessary to complete the plan. Once this is done, an analysis of potential disasters can begin. In this step, potential hazards are identified and vulnerability of the organization to disasters is assessed. A disaster response plan is established that includes the reduction/removal of hazardous situations. The final steps are plan implementation and review. The plan can be tested for efficacy through drills and mock disaster situations. It is critical to review and update the plan yearly.

There are several different types of disaster management plans, some more specific than others.

They are listed and briefly described below:
1. Emergency Action Plan – OSHA required, evacuation plans and emergency drills.
2. Business Continuity Plan – Business operation-specific, aimed at reducing losses and resuming productivity.
3. Risk Management Plan – Off-site effects of chemical exposures.
4. Emergency Response Plan – Immediate response to disasters.
5. Contingency Plan – General, designed to handle events not covered in other plans.
6. Federal Response Plan – Coordinates federal resources.
7. Spill Prevention, Control, and Countermeasures Plan – Deals with the prevention, control, and clean-up of oil spills.
8. Mutual Aid Plan – Plan for shared resources between other companies/firms.
9. Recovery Plan – Deals with repair and rebuilding post-disaster.
10. Emergency Management Plan – Plan for healthcare facilities.
11. All-Hazard Disaster Management Plan- General plan that is not hazard-specific.

Disaster/emergency response within the workplace

Once a disaster has occurred in the workplace, there are five basic stages of the response process. They are as follows (in order of operation): recognition that a disaster has occurred, notification of management and employees of the disaster, take steps to guarantee the immediate safety of employees, take steps to guarantee public safety, protection of property, and protection of the environment. The length of each stage depends on the scope of the disaster and how well previous stages were executed. Because people are the first priority of any disaster/emergency response, if there are any people left in harm's way, property and the environment cannot become a focus of protection.

Disaster recovery

Disaster recovery is the final stage of any disaster response and deals with the actions necessary to return the disaster site to normal. The recovery effort can be divided into two different periods: restoration and reconstruction/replacement. The restoration period is an immediate recovery step in which the area is made safe, utilities repaired, wreckage removed, and evacuees are allowed to return. The reconstruction/replacement period is a longer process where the disaster area is rebuilt and returned to its pre-disaster condition, both physically and economically. The reconstruction period can take many years, and is dependent on the degree of damage and availability of resources for reconstruction efforts. As a part of the disaster recovery process, steps should be taken to prevent a recurrence of the disaster in the future.

Incident Command System

The Incident Command System was developed by the Department of Homeland Security as a part of the National Incident Management System. It is a highly organized, hierarchical disaster management system that focuses on planning and organization, communication and delegation of responsibility, as well as response evaluation so that any disaster/emergency response effort runs as smoothly as possible. An Incident Commander (IC) is established as the person in charge. Safety officers, operations section officers, planning officers, and logistics officers are all appointed. These different officer positions are responsible for reporting back to the IC.

Terrorism

Terrorism is defined as the use of violence (or threat of violence) to frighten and coerce governments or societies into accepting the instigator's (terrorists) demands. The demands and goals of terrorists are often extreme and focused on areas with high population densities. This means that large companies can become potential targets of a terrorist attack. For this reason, when developing an emergency preparedness/disaster management plan, terrorist attacks should be included as a potential disaster. There are many different possible ways that terrorists can strike. Some examples are weapons of mass destruction, biological agents (i.e. bacteria, viruses, or toxins), nuclear and radiological incidents, incendiary devices, chemicals, and explosive devices.

Health impact assessment

Health impact assessment is a method of assessing the potential effects of a health policy or health program on the overall health of the population targeted by the policy or program. The purpose of health impact assessment is to maximize the benefits of health programs (in addition, of course, to minimizing the negative impact that the program may potentially have). There are typically 5 steps involved in the health impact assessment project; these steps include a screening process to ensure that the program is necessary or beneficial; scoping, which determines which population(s) will be impacted by the program; identification and assessment of all potential health impacts if the program is mandated; decision making and recommendations based on the assessment of potential impact; and evaluation and monitoring, which continues throughout the life of the program.

Nursing's Agenda for Health Care Reform from ANA

Nursing's Agenda for Health Care Reform – Encourages development of health care which gives patients the ability to get to good medical attention and help without it costing too much, and it encourages continual primary care. It fundamentally asks for vital medical attention to be found for everyone and for there to be a reorganized health care system that centers on patients, well-being and conditions so that they may get medical help in familiar, easy to get to places. It advocates providing for ongoing medical needs and insurance changes so that patients can use their coverage more easily. It asks for organizational assessment on public and private sectors regarding the use of resources, lowering expenses, and getting balanced and even reimbursement for each provider.

Organizing principles of care

When developing a model for patient-centered access to care, organizational considerations are important; in fact, organization is vital to any care plan model, but it is especially important to patient-centered care. Disorganization is a big part of the reason that the focus has fallen away from patient centered care. A hectic, disorganized, understaffed hospital emergency room is not able to provide patient-centered care even in the best of circumstances. The following organizing principles are necessary for an effective patient-centered access to care model: first, effective use of clinical resources and expertise; second, the alignment of care with patient needs and preferences; and third, services provided where they are needed.

Subacute care facilities

General—patients discharged to this level of care are stable and healing well but still require skilled care for such things as long-term intravenous treatments.

Chronic—chronic care facilities are for terminal and end-of-life patients that cannot be cared for in an at-home setting because of choice or complexity of care such as ventilator dependency.

Transitional—at this level, the patient still needs complex medical and nursing care, such as deep-wound management.

Long-term transitional—identifies a need for continued complex medical care that is expected to have an extended treatment time.

Continuum of care

The continuum of care refers to a series of services provided for patients or adults needing assistance across a span of time or through stages of change. The continuum of care may involve care practices used from the home, in the community, in a residential care facility, or another institution that provides care. This continuum meets the needs of the adult through stages of health or disability. By having a continuum of care, providers can better identify the needs of patients to provide and coordinate services as needed. For example, if a person needs to move from his home to a long-term care facility for residential treatment because of declining health, the continuum of care can give providers resources for helping the patient to make the transition. The care continuum ensures that all of the client's needs are met while making the transition. The process is tracked and evaluated to ensure competency and that services are complete.

The continuum of care is a series of care levels that meet patients where they are in terms of health. By identifying the level of the patient's needs, the continuum can guide clinicians for services. On one end is home care and intervention. This provides care for the patient in his home and identifies any additional needs. The next level might be outpatient services, in which the patient receives services at a healthcare center, but remains living at home. Beyond this level, the patient may need hospitalization or short-term care. This is more of an acute stage, but the patient does not need services for long. Following this, the patient might need inpatient care or assisted living services, this includes being monitored on a regular basis and no longer living at home. Finally, the end of the continuum involves high-need care, in which the patient requires intensive treatments because of a fragile state of health.

Published resources that are available regarding preventive care and health promotion

Of late, risk assessment, preventive medicine, and health promotion have become more and more important, and the focus of numerous studies. A study by Friede et al notes that almost 70% of illness, and the social, physical, psychological, and economical burden associated with it, is preventable. This is a staggering number, and highlights the importance of prevention. Healthy People 2000 and its latest version, Healthy People 2020, were published by the US Department of Health and Human Services, and they outline risks by age-group populations. A Guide to Clinical Preventive Services, also published by the DHHS, provides information for providers concerning burden of suffering, screening test accuracy, and efficiency of prevention for a number of illnesses associated with high morbidity and mortality.

Electronic medical records

Traditionally, the patient chart consisted of a clipboard with admission notes, progress notes, lab orders and results, and other patient information. There existed the potential for the chart to be lost or misplaced; in addition, serious errors in medication, patient identification, and ordering of tests could be attributed to a clinician's inability to decipher another clinician's handwritten notes. This one set of notes also made it difficult for other clinicians and allied health personnel in other departments to assess the patient. The advent of the electronic medical record helped to eliminate some of the problems associated with paper charts. Since the notes are entered into a computer system, illegible handwriting is no longer a source of error. The computerized system also allows clinicians in other areas of the hospital to access necessary information on patients, which improves the communication between clinicians and departments.

Measures taken by most hospitals to increase patient safety

Not all errors are preventable, but in the hospital setting, when errors can mean the difference between life and death, it is important that proper measures are undertaken to eliminate as many opportunities for error as possible. To prevent patient mix-ups, for instance, patients are required to wear an armband containing identification; the APRN or physician must check this identification against all orders to make sure that he or she has the correct patient. Hospital personnel should also wear an identifying tag or badge that contains the name of the employee, as well as his or her title and certification. This will help identify the employee not just to the patients but also to other employees. Another safeguard is the placement of signs on patient doors; these signs alert staff and other patients to any precautions that must be undertaken before entering the room, or while in the room (e.g., airborne precautions, fall precautions, elopement precautions).

Outcomes management

Outcomes management is defined by Wojner as "the enhancement of physiologic and psychosocial patient outcomes through development and implementation of exemplary health practices and services, as driven by outcomes assessment." An alternate definition of outcomes management, as stated by Ellwood, is "a technology of patient experience designed to help patients, payers, and providers make rational medical care-related choices based on better insight into the effects of these choices on the patient's life." Although the 2 men had different definitions for outcome management, the line of thinking is the same, and that is the importance of a link between patient outcomes and quality control measures used to ensure that the best possible outcomes are arrived at as often as possible.

The outcomes management quality model has 4 separate phases. The first phase includes the identification of long-term outcomes for the patient in order to gauge the length of the time of care and to set a starting point. Another part of phase 1 is the selection of instruments to be used for the longitudinal study; in other words, what instruments are going to be used to determine the long-term care outcomes. These instruments typically assess quality of life, functional status, and patient satisfaction. Phase 1 also includes the identification of intermediate outcomes, which may include setbacks in the patient care process. The identification of variances that lead to setbacks in care (such as laboratory errors or physician errors) is also a part of phase 1. The last important part of phase 1 is the creation of a population database.

Phase 2 of the outcomes management quality model includes the review of both traditional practice and existing literature. The overall purpose or goal of phase 2 of the model is the development of interdisciplinary practice standards. During phase 2, the members of the interdisciplinary team will gather to discuss and negotiate existing and proposed practice standards. The protocols, pathways, and order sets that are designed and formulated during this period are all considered to be "structured care methodologies" (SCMs). These SCMs will be used on the patient cohort population. Once the interdisciplinary team has decided on a set of SCMs for the cohort, the entire initiative can be standardized.

Phase 3 of the outcomes management quality model is the actual implementation of the structured care methodologies within the patient cohort population. These newly instituted structured care methodologies become the standard of practice, and once the members of the interdisciplinary team and other pertinent staff members are educated about the new practices, data collection can be initiated. If the new practices are expensive (if they require expensive equipment and maintenance, or more supplies, or more billable hours initially), the interdisciplinary team should conduct a cost-benefit analysis, the obvious benefits being that length of stay, number of complications, and number of patient readmissions will be reduced as a result of the new practices.

Phase 4, the final phase of the outcomes management quality model, involves a thorough, in-depth analysis of the interdisciplinary data that have accumulated during the course of the outcomes management initiative process. Once the data have been analyzed, the interdisciplinary team should meet to discuss whether certain practices or structured care methodologies should be revised to optimize outcomes management. If the team does identify practices that need revision, the initiative will return to phase 2. After this discussion, the interdisciplinary team should discuss any new questions or hypotheses that are related to outcomes management in order to perhaps begin another initiative.

Practice Test

Practice Questions

1. Which of the following techniques should be used when interviewing an elderly woman?
   a. Speak quickly to get through a focused assessment before the woman tires
   b. Speak in a quiet and calming tone so that the woman does not become agitated
   c. Speak loudly and clearly so that the woman can hear you
   d. Perform the entire interview in front of the primary caregiver

2. A 77-year-old male patient has increasing dementia with short-term memory loss and symptoms that fluctuate frequently. The patient experiences visual hallucination and exhibits muscle rigidity and tremors. These symptoms are characteristic of which type of non-Alzheimer's dementia?
   a. Dementia with Lewy bodies
   b. Frontotemporal dementia
   c. Normal pressure hydrocephalus
   d. Parkinson's dementia

3. Who determines an APRN's right to write prescriptions?
   a. Standards of Practice
   b. The American Nursing Association
   c. The state where the APRN is practicing
   d. The Drug Enforcement Agency

4. A 40-year-old female hospitalized for severe exacerbation of asthma has been treated for 6 days with albuterol by small volume nebulizer, oral theophylline, and IV methylprednisolone. The patient's blood gases have stabilized. When discontinuing the IV steroid in preparation for discharge, the acute care nurse practitioner should order:
   a. Inhaled steroid, such as Azmacort, only
   b. Oral prednisone 20 mg daily for one week and then Azmacort
   c Oral prednisone in decreasing doses
   d. Oral prednisone in decreasing doses and inhaled steroid, such as Azmacort

5. Which of the following statements is CORRECT about Medicaid?
   a. Everyone who falls below the federal poverty line is eligible to receive Medicaid
   b. The state is allowed to require that recipients pay a small copayment
   c. Recipients of Medicaid are not supposed to pay anything towards their medical care
   d. Though it is both a federal and state plan, only the state government is responsible for supervision of the program

6. A woman complains of a history of nausea and burning, stabbing epigastric pain which is relieved for short periods by antacids or intake of food. The patient denies NSAID use but is a heavy smoker. A urea breath test is positive. Which of the following treatment protocols is most common?

    a. Histamine-2 blocker plus bismuth plus tetracycline

    b. Proton pump inhibitor only

    c. Proton pump inhibitor plus tetracycline

    d. Proton pump inhibitor plus clarithromycin and amoxicillin/metronidazole

7. A patient who receives multiple transfusions with citrated blood products must be monitored closely for:

    a. Hyponatremia

    b. Hypomagnesemia

    c. Hypokalemia

    d. Hypocalcemia

8. Negligence is:

    a. Not acting in a way that a reasonable and prudent nurse would, and the patient was harmed

    b. Acting in a way that is against the law, when the patient has been harmed

    c. Not taking the appropriate preventative measures that another nurse would, to the detriment of the patient

    d. Not giving appropriate medical care to a patient

9. An incidence of which of the following conditions requires mandatory reporting to the CDC?

    a. Influenza

    b. Lyme disease

    c. Hepatitis E

    d. Methicillin-resistant Staphylococcus aureus infection

10. Which of the following arterial blood gas (ABG) findings is consistent with metabolic acidosis in an adult?

    a. HCO_3 <22 mEq/L and pH <7.35

    b. HCO_3 >26 mEq/L and pH >7.45

    c. $PaCO_2$ 35–45 mm Hg and PaO_2 ≥80 mg Hg

    d. $PaCO_2$ >55 mm Hg and PaO_2 <60

11. A thin young adult comes into the emergency room with a sudden onset of right-sided chest pain and shortness of breath following a run. What do you suspect?

    a. Myocardial infarction

    b. Aortic dissection

    c. Asthma flare

    d. Spontaneous pneumothorax

12. A patient with severe type 1 diabetes mellitus refuses all treatment because of religious convictions. Which of the following is the most appropriate action?

    a. Provide the patient with facts about the disease, treatments, and prognosis.

    b. Ask family members to intervene.

    c. Remind the patient that he will die without treatment.

    d. Refer the patient to a psychologist.

13. A young woman presents in the emergency room with sudden shortness of breath, coughing, and slight chest pain. She is on the birth control pill and just returned home from a car trip several hours away. What tests should you order?

    a. ABG, ECG, chest x-ray, and echocardiogram

    b. CBC, pulmonary function test, stress test

    c. ECG, cardiac enzymes, stress test

    d. Sputum culture, CBC, pulmonary function test

14. When irrigating a wound, what wound irrigation pressure is needed to effectively cleanse the wound while avoiding trauma?

    a. <4 psi

    b. 20–30 psi

    c. 10–15 psi

    d. >15 psi

15. A thyroid panel comes back with the following results: elevated TSH, low free T4, and low free T3. What is the diagnosis?

    a. Hyperthyroidism

    b. Subclinical hypothyroidism

    c. Primary hypothyroidism

    d. Subclinical hyperthyroidism

16. When the nurse practitioner enters the room of a patient whose death is imminent, the daughter states, "I can't stay in the room when Dad dies! I can't stand the thought!" Which of the following is the best response?

    a. "You will regret it if you don't."

    b. "Your father would want you with him."

    c. "I'll stay with him, and you can come and go as you feel comfortable."

    d. "Is there someone else who can stay with him?"

17. A patient has chest pain, dyspnea, and hypotension. A 12-lead ECG shows atrial rates of 250 with regular ventricular rates of 100. P waves are saw-toothed (referred to as F waves), QRS shape and duration (0.4 to 0.11 seconds) is normal, PR interval is hard to calculate because of F waves, and the P:QRS ratio is 2–4:1. Which of the following diagnoses fits this profile?

    a. Premature atrial contraction

    b. Premature junctional contraction

    c. Atrial fibrillation

    d. Atrial flutter

18. What is the antibiotic of choice in a patient with syphilis, who reports an allergy to penicillin?
    a. Doxycycline 100 mg PO BID x 14 days
    b. Ofloxacin 400 mg PO BID x 14 days
    c. Ceftriaxone 250 mg IM x 1 dose
    d. Metronidazole 500 mg PO BID x 14 days

19. Which of the following communication approaches is most effective to facilitate communication with a patient who has global aphasia?
    a. Speak slowly and clearly, facing the patient.
    b. Use letter boards.
    c. Ask yes/no questions.
    d. Use pictures, diagrams, and gestures.

20. A 44-year-old obese woman recovering from a femoropopliteal bypass develops sudden onset of dyspnea with chest pain on inspiration, cough, and fever of 39°C. An S_4 gallop rhythm is present. The ECG shows tachycardia and nonspecific changes in ST and T waves. The most likely diagnosis is:
    a. Myocardial infarction
    b. Pulmonary embolism
    c. Pneumonia
    d. Sepsis

21. Which drug that is used for the treatment of coronary artery disease should be avoided in patients with asthma?
    a. Spironolactone
    b. Losartan
    c. Propranolol
    d. Captopril

22. When determining the burden of proof for acts of negligence, how would risk management classify willfully providing inadequate care while disregarding the safety and security of another?
    a. Negligent conduct
    b. Gross negligence
    c. Contributory negligence
    d. Comparative negligence

23. Which antibiotic should be avoided in patients taking theophylline?
    a. Doxycycline
    b. Erythromycin
    c. Vancomycin
    d. Penicillin

24. A 25-year-old patient with multiple fractures from an auto accident develops hypoxia, dyspnea, precordial chest pain, tachycardia, and thick milky sputum. Auscultation of the lungs shows crackles and wheezes. The patient complains of headache and has a fever of 40°C. Which of the following interventions should be done first?
    a. High-flow oxygen
    b. Corticosteroids (IV)
    c. Vasopressors
    d. Morphine

25. In patients taking valproic acid for seizure disorder, serum levels should be maintained at:
    a. 50 to 100 mcg/mL
    b. 20 to 80 mcg/mL
    c. 10 to 20 mcg/mL
    d. 4 to 12 mcg/mL

26. When the nurse practitioner is conducting medication reconciliation, the patient's list of current medications includes the following: Lasix®, metolazone, aminophylline, and doxapram. The nurse believes this list probably indicates
    a. polypharmacy.
    b. inaccurate reporting.
    c. accurate reporting.
    d. poor medical management.

27. A patient is hospitalized for a myocardial infarction and exhibits increased preload, increased afterload, and decreased contractility with decreased cardiac output and increased systemic vascular resistance. BP is 84/40 and pulse 124 bpm, thready, and irregular. The patient has tachypnea, chest pain, basilar rales, and pallor. The most likely diagnosis is:
    a. Cardiogenic shock
    b. Pulmonary embolism
    c. Heart failure
    d. Atrial fibrillation

28. Which of the following sensory changes associated with aging has the most impact on older adults?
    a. Hearing deficit
    b. Vision deficit
    c. Decreased taste and smell
    d. Decreased sense of touch (vibration, temperature, pain)

29. An HIV-positive patient has experienced a recent drop in CD4 count to 190. She has developed a fever with general malaise and abdominal pain, and examination shows hepatosplenomegaly. Differential diagnoses should include:
    a. Pneumocystis jiroveci pneumonia, bacterial pneumonia, and TB
    b. Toxoplasmosis, herpes encephalitis, and CNS lymphoma
    c. Histoplasmosis, Mycobacterium avium complex, and bacillary peliosis
    d. TB, non-Hodgkin's lymphoma, and bacillary angiomatosis

30. With the Braden scale to assess risk for developing pressure sores, the patient scores 1 to 3 in all six assessment areas with a total score of 14. What is the patient's risk?
    a. High risk, poor prognosis
    b. Breakpoint for risk, moderate prognosis
    c. Minimal risk, excellent prognosis
    d. No risk

31. An 80-year-old male has had post-herpetic neuralgia for 11 months, but pain is increasingly intractable despite his taking 10 hydrocodone tablets daily. He has coronary stents in place and takes warfarin. The patient is weak, somnolent, and lethargic, and eats and sleeps poorly. Modifying his pain management should include:
    a. Weaning patient from hydrocodone and starting gabapentin in slowly increasing doses
    b. Discontinuing hydrocodone and starting morphine pump
    c. Weaning patient from hydrocodone and starting biofeedback
    d. Lowering the dose of hydrocodone and supplementing with NSAIDs

32. A 76-year-old male is recovering from surgery but exhibits sudden onset of confusion with fluctuating inattention, disorganized thinking, and altered level of consciousness. Which of the following assessment tools is most indicated?
    a. Mini-mental state exam (MMSE)
    b. Mini-Cog
    c. Confusion assessment method (CAM)
    d. Geriatric depression scale (GDS)

33. When forced expiratory volume in one second (FEV_1) is markedly more reduced than the reduction in forced vital capacity (FVC), the patient is probably experiencing:
    a. Restriction of maximal lung expansion
    b. Airway obstruction
    c. Depressed respiratory center
    d. Limitation in neurological impulses to the muscles of respiration

34. A 70-year-old female with Alzheimer's and a history of falls is admitted to the unit with pneumonitis after a seven-hour wait in the emergency department. The patient is agitated, restless, and repeatedly says "I'm hungry." The nurse's first priority should be to
    a. assess diet needs and order food.
    b. institute a fall-prevention program.
    c. review all medications.
    d. assess cognitive abilities.

35. A patient with a score of 10 on the Glasgow coma scale is classified as:
    a. Comatose
    b. Severe head injury
    c. Moderate head injury
    d. Mild head injury

36. A patient's laboratory tests show that the TSH is 14 mU/mL, free T4 is 3.5 µg/dL and free T3 is 100 ng/dL. These findings indicate
    a. normal values.
    b. hypothyroidism.
    c. hyperthyroidism.
    d. Hashimoto's thyroiditis.

37. A patient with bone metastasis from prostate cancer is to be treated with zoledronic acid (Reclast®, Zometa®). Which laboratory test(s) must be done prior to initiating treatment?
    a. Serum creatinine/creatinine clearance
    b. Blood urea nitrogen (BUN)
    c. Complete blood count (CBC)
    d. Electrolyte panel

38. A 69-year-old female hospitalized for a fractured hip is being evaluated for comorbidities. The most common comorbidity for hospitalized patients ages 65 to 80 is
    a. fluid and electrolyte imbalance.
    b. COPD.
    c. anemia.
    d. hypertension.

39. A 45-year-old male has renal calculi. He has passed one stone, but ultrasound shows multiple stones present in the urinary tract. Stone analysis shows the stone is calcium-containing. In addition to analgesia and antispasmodics, which medication is indicated?
    a. Indomethacin
    b. Allopurinol and Vitamin B6
    c. Alpha-mercato-propionyl-glycine (aMPG) and captopril
    d. Hydrochlorothiazide

40. When prescribing an oral anti-diabetic agent for an older patient, the patient's initial dose should be
    a. the same as the usual dose for a younger adult.
    b. 25% of the usual dose.
    c. 50% of the usual dose.
    d. 75% of the usual dose.

41. A 56-year-old female has pain and swelling of the small joints of the hands and wrist. Which test(s) should the acute care nurse practitioner order to confirm a diagnosis of rheumatoid arthritis?
    a. Rheumatoid factor (RF) and anti-citrullinated protein antibody (ACPA)
    b. RF and erythrocyte sedimentation rate (ESR)
    c. C-reactive protein (CRP) and RF
    d. Synovial fluid analysis, ESR, and CRP

42. A 78-year-old patient is hospitalized with severe dehydration from influenza. Which type of precaution is indicated when caring for the patient?
    a. Use personal protective equipment, including gown and gloves for all contact.
    b. Wear a mask while caring for patient.
    c. Wear a mask and gloves for all contact with patient.
    d. Use a ≥N95 respirator while caring for patient.

43. A patient has a chronic leg ulcer covered with black eschar and is to have chemical debridement with collagenase. Preparation includes:
    a. Thoroughly drying the eschar and surrounding skin
    b. Applying topical antibiotic
    c. Scrubbing the wound with hexachlorophene
    d. Cross-hatching the upper layers of the eschar

44. A 36-year-old female was injured in a fall when drunk. CT shows contusion on the left side of the brain. The patient responds lethargically to verbal commands and shows some confusion and restlessness. Vital signs: BP 154/76, pulse 68, and respirations 28. Previous records indicate her normal BP was 128/70, pulse 76, and respirations 16. The change in VS is most likely an indication of:
    a. Increasing intracranial pressure
    b. Stress response
    c. Ethanol intoxication
    d. Delirium tremens

45. Which of the following is the best documentation of the behavior of a difficult patient?
    a. "Patient is belligerent and uncooperative."
    b. "Patient is spitting at nurses, throwing magazines, and refusing to get out of bed for therapy."
    c. "Patient appears to dislike nurses and other care providers."
    d. "Patient believes staff members are going to hurt her."

46. A 75-year-old male is receiving warfarin after the insertion of an aortic stent for aortic aneurysm. The patient states he usually takes a number of vitamins and herbal preparations. Which of the following should the patient avoid?
    a. St. John's wort
    b. Melatonin
    c. Echinacea
    d. Vitamin B complex

47. A retrospective attempt to determine the cause of an event, often a sentinel event such as an unexpected death, is:
    a. T-test
    b. Regression analysis
    c. Tracer methodology
    d. Root cause analysis

48. A 72-year-old female on Medicare is being discharged home with a healing burn on her left arm that she is unable to care for independently because of arthritis. She requires dressing changes every 3 days. She depends on public transportation and walks with difficulty. The bus stop is two blocks from her house. Her 12-year-old granddaughter lives with her. The best solution is:
    a. Transferring the patient to an extended care facility
    b. Providing treatment on an outpatient basis at the hospital clinic
    c. Teaching the woman's 12-year-old granddaughter to do the dressing changes
    d. Making a referral to a home health agency to provide in-home care

49. If all patients who develop urinary infections with urinary catheters are evaluated per urine culture and sensitivities for microbial resistance, but only those patients with clinically evident infections are included, this is an example of:
    a. Information bias
    b. Selection bias
    c. Compliance bias
    d. Admission bias

50. A 68-year-old male has an asynchronous pacemaker and has been experiencing cardiac palpitations, headache, and anxiety, general malaise, pain in the jaw and chest, and unexplained weakness with pulsations evident in the neck and abdomen. The most likely cause is:
    a. Broken pacemaker wires
    b. Dislodged pacemaker wires
    c. Myocardial infarction
    d. Pacemaker syndrome

Answers and Explanations

1. C: Speaking quickly or quietly may make it difficult for the woman to hear you. If possible, the interview should be performed outside of the presence of the primary caregiver so you can properly screen for elder abuse. If this is not possible, at least perform that part of the screening while the patient is alone. When interviewing an elderly woman, you should speak in a clear voice at an adequate volume, while facing the patient. Watch for signs that she is tiring or becoming stressed and adjust your technique accordingly, or take a break if necessary.

2. A: These symptoms are characteristic of dementia with Lewy bodies. Cognitive and physical decline is similar to Alzheimer's, but symptoms may fluctuate frequently. This form of dementia may include visual hallucinations, muscle rigidity, and tremors. Frontotemporal dementia may cause marked changes in personality and behavior and is characterized by difficulty using and understanding language. Normal pressure hydrocephalus is characterized by ataxia, memory loss, and urinary incontinence. Parkinson's dementia may involve impaired decision making and difficulty concentrating, learning new material, understanding complex language, and sequencing as well as inflexibility and short- or long-term memory loss.

3. C: The ability to write prescriptions is dictated by the scope of practice, which is set by the state in which the nurse is practicing.

4. D: Patients receiving oral or intravenous steroids should be prescribed oral prednisone in decreasing doses while initiating inhaled steroids. Severe episodes of asthma may occur with withdrawal of oral or IV steroids when switching to inhaled aerosol, so combining inhaled treatment with decreasing doses can help prevent adrenal suppression, which results in acute exacerbation of symptoms. Patients should use a metered-dose inhaler (MDI) with a reservoir device or a formulation with a spacing tube (such as Azmacort) and rinse the mouth thoroughly after inhaling to prevent thrush.

5. B: Medicaid is not always completely free for those who receive aid. Though they cannot bill recipients for medical care, the state is allowed by the federal government to charge a small co-pay. Not everyone who lives below the federal poverty guidelines will qualify for Medicaid. Medicaid is overseen by both the state and federal governments.

6. D: These symptoms are consistent with a duodenal ulcer, and the positive urea breath test indicates a *Helicobacter pylori* infection, which is usually treated with a proton pump inhibitor plus clarithromycin and amoxicillin/metronidazole. About 90% of duodenal ulcers are associated with *H. pylori* infection. *H. pylori* weakens the mucosa and results in hypersecretion of gastric acid. Eating may increase pain with gastric ulcers but usually relieves pain with duodenal ulcers. Smoking increases the risk of peptic ulcer disease, and use of NSAIDs increases risk of serious complications, such as bleeding or perforation.

7. D: Patients who receive multiple transfusions with citrated blood products must be carefully monitored for hypocalcemia. Calcium is important for transmitting nerve impulses and regulating muscle contraction and relaxation, including the myocardium. Calcium

activates enzymes that stimulate chemical reactions and has a role in coagulation of blood. Values include:

- Normal values: 8.2 to 10.2 mg/dL.
- Hypocalcemia: <8.2 mg/dL. Critical value: <7 mg/dL.
- Hypercalcemia: >10.2 mg/dL. Critical value: >12 mg/dL.

Symptoms include tetany, tingling, seizures, altered mental status, and ventricular tachycardia. Treatment is calcium replacement and vitamin D.

8. A: The definition of negligence is when a medical professional acts in a way that a reasonable person of the same education and skill level would not, and this action results in patient harm. Disloyalty, acting in an illegal manner, or not acting at all to prevent a patient from being harmed is called malpractice.

9. B: Lyme disease requires mandatory reporting while reporting of the other diseases is voluntary. The CDC maintains a reportable disease list, which is upgraded and revised as necessary and reissued July 1 of each year. Each state also maintains a reportable disease list, which may or may not be identical with that of the CDC, so the nurse must be familiar with all reportable disease requirements. Much data at the state and local level is confidential name-based information, but data collected at the CDC is without names or personal identifying information. Some states require reporting of hospital-acquired infections.

10. A: HCO_3 <22 mEq/L and pH <7.35 are consistent with metabolic acidosis, which may result from severe diarrhea, starvation, DKA, kidney failure, and aspirin toxicity. Symptoms may include headache, altered consciousness, agitation, lethargy, and coma. Cardiac dysrhythmias and Kussmaul respiration are common. Other readings:

- HCO_3 >26 mEq/L and pH >7.45 are consistent with metabolic alkalosis.
- $PaCO_2$ 35–45 mm Hg and PaO_2 ≥80 mg Hg are normal adult readings.
- D. $PaCO_2$ >55 mm Hg and PaO_2 <60 are consistent with acute respiratory failure in a previously healthy adult.

11. D: Young, thin males are particularly prone to spontaneous pneumothorax, especially following exercise. Shortness of breath would not be present in patients having an aortic dissection, and chest pain would be on the left side if they were having an MI. Asthma generally does not cause chest pain.

12. A: Patients have a right to refuse treatment for religious or other personal reasons, so the most appropriate action is to simply provide the patient with factual information about the disease, treatments, and prognosis in a neutral manner, without trying to coerce or frighten the patient. In some cases, patients may change their minds when presented with information, but the nurse should remain supportive regardless of the patient's decision. Asking the family to intervene is not appropriate and refusal of treatment alone does not suggest the need for referral to a psychologist.

13. A: Given her history, you should immediately suspect that she has a pulmonary embolus, or a blood clot that passed into the lung tissue. You should order an ABG to assess oxygenation, and an ECG and chest x-ray to rule out other causative conditions.

14. C: Wounds should be irrigated with pressures of 10 to 15 psi. An irrigation pressure of <4 psi does not adequately cleanse a wound, and pressures >15 psi can result in trauma to the wound, interfering with healing. A mechanical irrigation device is more effective for irrigation than a bulb syringe, which delivers about ≤2 psi. A 250 mL squeeze bottle supplies about 4.5 psi, adequate for low-pressure cleaning. A 35-mL syringe with a 19-gauge needle provides about 8 psi.

15. C: When the TSH is elevated, it is an indication that the thyroid is in a sluggish (i.e., hypothyroid) state and needs higher amounts of TSH to stimulate production of the thyroid hormones. In primary hypothyroidism, both levels of free T4 and free T3 are low. In cases of subclinical hypothyroidism, free T3 and free T4 are not affected, and their levels remain within the normal range.

16. C: The nurse practitioner should remain supportive and nonjudgmental. "I'll stay with him, and you can come and go as you feel comfortable" supports the daughter's stated desire while still leaving open the opportunity for her to spend time with her father during the death vigil. People react in very different ways to death, and many people have never seen a deceased person and may be very frightened. While many people find comfort in being with a dying friend or family member, this should never be imposed on anyone.

17. D:

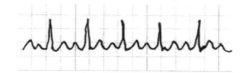

Atrial flutter (AF) occurs when the atrial rate is faster (usually 250–400 beats per minute) than the atrioventricular (AV) node conduction rate so not all of the beats are conducted into the ventricles (ventricular rate 75–150). The beats are effectively blocked at the AV node, preventing ventricular fibrillation although some extra ventricular impulses may go through. AF is caused by the same conditions that cause atrial fibrillation: coronary artery disease, valvular disease, pulmonary disease, heavy alcohol ingestion, and cardiac surgery. Treatment includes:

- Cardioversion if condition is unstable.
- Medications to slow ventricular rate and conduction through AV node: Cardizem®, Calan®.
- Medications to convert to sinus rhythm: Corvert®, Cardioquin®, Norpace®, Cordarone®.

18. A: Except for neurosyphilis, the primary treatment should be penicillin G 2.4 million units IM for one dose. In patients who are allergic to penicillin, the treatment of choice is doxycycline 100 mg PO twice a day for 14 days OR tetracycline 500 mg PO four times a day for 14 days. Pregnant patients are an exception; they should still be given penicillin after undergoing desensitization.

19. D: Aphasia is the loss of ability to use and/or understand written and spoken language because of damage to the speech center of the brain caused by brain tumors, brain injury, and stroke. Global aphasia is characterized by difficulty understanding and producing language in speaking, reading, and writing although patients may understand gestures. The

nurse can use pictures, diagrams, and gestures to convey meaning. Picture charts are also useful. The speech pathologist should assess patients with aphasia and provide guidance in communicating with them.

20. B: Although symptoms of pulmonary embolism may vary widely depending on the size and location of the embolus, dyspnea, inspirational chest pain, cough, fever, S4 sound, tachycardia, and non-specific ECG changes in ST and T waves are common. Risk factors include obesity, recent surgery, history of deep vein thrombosis, and inactivity. Treatment includes oxygen, IV fluids, dobutamine for hypotension, analgesia for anxiety, and medications as indicated (digitalis, diuretic, antiarrhythmic). Intubation and mechanical ventilation may be required. Percutaneous filter may be placed in the inferior vena cava to prevent more emboli from reaching lungs.

21. C: Propranolol is a beta-blocker and reduces myocardial demand for oxygen. It also can cause bronchospasm and should be avoided in patients who have any form of bronchospastic disease, such as asthma.

22. B: Gross negligence. Negligence indicates that *proper care* has not been provided, based on established standards. *Reasonable care* uses rationale for decision making in relation to providing care. Types of negligence:
- Negligent conduct indicates that an individual failed to provide reasonable care or to protect/assist another, based on standards and expertise.
- Gross negligence is willfully providing inadequate care while disregarding the safety and security of another.
- Contributory negligence involves the injured party contributing to his/her own harm.
- Comparative negligence attempts to determine what percentage amount of negligence is attributed to each individual involved.

23. B: Erythromycin lessens theophylline's effectiveness and should not be prescribed in a patient who is taking theophylline. Consider an alternate antibiotic.

24. A: These symptoms are consistent with fat embolism syndrome (FES), which may cause rapid acute pulmonary edema and ARDS, so the patient should be immediately provided with high-flow oxygen. Controlled-volume ventilation with positive end-expiratory pressure (PEEP) may be indicated to prevent/treat pulmonary edema. Corticosteroids may reduce inflammation of the lungs and reduce cerebral edema. Vasopressors prevent hypotension and interstitial pulmonary edema. Morphine with a benzodiazepine may be indicated for patients who require artificial ventilation.

25. A: The therapeutic serum levels for valproic acid is between 50 and 100 mcg/mL. Clonazepam therapeutic serum levels are between 20 and 80 ng/mL. Carbamazepine should be maintained at serum levels of 4 to 12 mcg/mL, and phenytoin should be maintained at serum levels of 10 to 20 mcg/mL.

26. A: Since Lasix® and metolazone are both diuretics and aminophylline and doxapram are both methylxanthines, this list probably indicates polypharmacy. Older adults are especially at risk for polypharmacy—taking too many drugs—because of taking the same drug under generic and brand names, taking drugs for one condition but contraindicated for another, and taking drugs that are not compatible. Reasons for polypharmacy include multiple

prescriptions from different doctors; forgetfulness; confusion; failure to report current medications; the use of supplemental, over-the-counter, and herbal preparations in addition to prescribed medications; and failure of healthcare providers to adequately educate the patient.

27. A: These symptoms are consistent with cardiogenic shock. Cardiogenic shock has 3 characteristics: Increased preload, increased afterload, and decreased contractibility. Together these result in a decreased cardiac output and an increase in systemic vascular resistance (SVR) to compensate and protect vital organs. This results in an increase of afterload in the left ventricle with increased need for oxygen. As the cardiac output continues to decrease, tissue perfusion decreases, coronary artery perfusion decreases, fluid backs up, and the left ventricle fails to adequately pump the blood, resulting in pulmonary edema and right ventricular failure.

28. B: Older adults are most impacted by deteriorating vision (presbyopia, cataracts), which prevents them from reading and navigating safely. Most people older than 60 require glasses. People may be less sensitive to color differences (particularly blues and greens), and night vision decreases. Hearing impairment (impacted cerumen, presbycusis) may require periodic cleaning of the ears or hearing aids. Taste and smell usually remain fairly intact although smell of airborne chemicals may be less acute, and taste buds begin to atrophy around age 60, affecting the ability to taste sweet and salt especially. The sense of touch is usually somewhat reduced in older adults.

29. C: Fever, malaise, abdominal pain, and hepatosplenomegaly in an HIV-positive patient with CD4 count <200 may result from histoplasmosis, Mycobacterium avium complex, and bacillary peliosis. Fever, cough, and dyspnea may indicate Pneumocystis jiroveci pneumonia, bacterial pneumonia, and TB. Fever, headache, neck pain, and altered mental status may indicate toxoplasmosis, herpes encephalitis, and CNS lymphoma. Fever with asymmetric or unilateral lymphadenopathy may indicate TB, non-Hodgkin's lymphoma, and bacillary angiomatosis.

30. B: Breakpoint for risk, moderate prognosis. Six assessment areas include sensory perception, moisture, activity, mobility, usual nutrition pattern, and friction and sheer. The first four categories are scored from 1 (worst) to 4 (best) and the last category (friction and sheer) is scored from 1 to 3. The scores for all six items are totaled and a risk assigned according to the number.
23: (Best score) excellent prognosis, very minimal risk
≤16: Breakpoint for risk of pressure ulcer (will vary somewhat for different populations)
6: (Worst score) prognosis very poor, strong likelihood of developing pressure ulcers

31. A: Post-herpetic neuralgia is a chronic pain condition that responds poorly to opioids and is better treated with anticonvulsants, such as gabapentin. Tricyclic antidepressants are also used but may have severe side effects in the elderly. Because the patient has been on high doses of hydrocodone, he may experience withdrawal with abrupt discontinuation of the drug, so the dose should be decreased by one tablet every 2 to 3 days while gabapentin is started at a low dose and slowly increased to reduce incidence of side effects. Morphine pumps and NSAIDs are usually avoided with warfarin and are often ineffective.

32. C: CAM: Assesses development of delirium. Factors indicative of delirium include Onset: Acute change in mental status.

Attention: Inattentive, stable, or fluctuating.

Thinking: Disorganized, rambling conversation, switching topics, illogical.

Level of consciousness: Altered, ranging from alert to coma.

Orientation: Disoriented (person, place, time).

Memory: Impaired.

Perceptual disturbances: Hallucinations, illusions.

Psychomotor abnormalities: Agitation (tapping, picking, moving) or retardation (staring, not moving).

Sleep-wake cycle: Awake at night and sleepy in the daytime.

MMSE and Mini-Cog are used to assess evidence of dementia or short-term memory loss, often associated with Alzheimer's disease. GDS is a self-assessment tool to identify older adults with depression.

33. B: Airway obstruction often results in FEV_1 that is more reduced than FVC because the air is trapped and cannot be readily expelled in one second. Normally, FEV_1 is about 80% of vital capacity with most of the remaining air expelled by 3 seconds (FEV_3). Proportional reduction of both FEV_1 and FVC indicate reduced lung expansion. Depression of respiratory centers results from anesthesia or sedation. Limitation in neurological impulses results from damage to the brain or spinal cord.

34. A: The first priority should be to attend to the patient's comfort needs by assessing diet needs, including food allergies, and ordering food. Because the patient has a history of falls, the nurse practitioner should institute a program of fall prevention, assessing the best methods to prevent injury to the patient. The nurse should then review all medications to ensure that no ongoing medical needs are overlooked, as patients may not provide full information in the emergency department. Cognitive abilities are best assessed when the patient is comfortable and rested.

35. C: A score of 10 on the Glasgow Coma Scale (GCS) indicates a moderate head injury. GCS measures the depth and duration of coma or impaired level of consciousness and is used for postoperative/brain injury assessment. The GCS measures three parameters—best eye response, best verbal response, and best motor response—with a total possible score that ranges from 3 to 15. Injuries/conditions are classified according to the total score:

- 3–8 coma
- ≥8 severe head injury
- 9–12 moderate head injury
- 13–15 mild head injury

36. B: These laboratory findings indicate hypothyroidism, which is characterized by increased TSH, decreased free T4, and normal free T3. Normal values for an older adult:

TSH: 0.32–5.0 mU/mL.

Free T4: 4.5–12 µg/dL

Free T3: 75–200 ng/dL.

Hyperthyroidism is characterized by decreased TSH (<0.30), increased free T4 and increased T3. Additional tests may be indicated for those with comorbidities and multiple medications. Thyroid autoantibody tests are used to help diagnose Hashimoto's thyroiditis.

37. A: Because zoledronic acid may result in decreased renal function in acute renal failure, a serum creatinine and calculation of creatinine clearance should be done before every dose. Zoledronic acid is contraindicated with creatinine clearance <35 mL/min or with

severe renal impairment. Additional treatments are withheld if renal deterioration occurs and not resumed until creatinine is within 10% of baseline value. Normal CC values: Adult male: 97–137 mL/min: Adult female: 88–128 mL/min. During treatment, patients should receive calcium (500 mg) and vitamin D (400 IU) supplements daily unless the patient has hypercalcemia.

38. D: The most common comorbidities (with approximate percentages) for those hospitalized include:

Hypertension: 30% COPD: 12% Diabetes: 12% Fluid/electrolyte imbalance: 12% Iron deficiency/anemia: 8%	CHF: 6% Hypothyroidism: 6% Depression/bipolar disorder: 5% Neurological disorder: 4% Obesity: 4%

Comorbidities vary according to age. In those under 18 and over 80, fluid and electrolyte disorders from dehydration or excess fluids predominate while hypertension is most common for those over 18. Diabetes is the next most common disorder for those under 80.

39. D: Thiazides, such as hydrochlorothiazide, are indicated to increase reabsorption of calcium with calcium-containing renal calculi. Allopurinol and vitamin B6 are used with oxalate-containing stones. Alpha-mercato-propionyl-glycine (aMPG) and captopril are used with cystine-containing stones if increasing hydration and alkalinization is ineffective. Indomethacin is used with allopurinol to maintain uric acid levels. Alkalinizing agents, such as Polycitra and Allopurinol, are used with uric acid stones. Additional medications can include antibiotics if infection occurs. Some patients may require opioids, such as morphine, to control pain.

40. C: 50%.

Problems associated with older adults and different types of drugs	
Anti-diabetics	Oral anti-diabetic agents should be started at 50% of the usual dose because of the danger of hypoglycemia. First generation drugs should be avoided. Glucotrol® has fewer side effects than Diabeta®.
Antidepressants	Antidepressants are associated with excess sedation, so typical doses are only 16–33% of a younger adult's dose. SSRIs are safest, but Prozac® may cause anorexia, anxiety, and insomnia so should be avoided.
Anticoagulants	Anticoagulants may cause severe bleeding in those over 65. Warfarin should be used with care and at a lower dose if total protein or albumin concentration is low.

41. A: Tests for diagnosis of rheumatoid arthritis in the presence of joint involvement of the small joints (fingers, wrists) or large joints (elbows, hips, knees) includes primarily RF and ACPA. ESR and CRP may also show elevation but are less specific. Diagnosis is usually made if 4 of 7 positive symptoms for RA are present: morning stiffness >1 hour, ≥2 involved joints with involvement of wrists, or finger joints >6 weeks, bilateral and symmetrical

involvement, presence of rheumatoid nodules, joint destruction on x-ray, and positive RF or ACPA.

42. B: Influenza requires droplet precautions, using a mask.

Contact	Use personal protective equipment (PPE), including gown and gloves, for all contacts with the patient or patient's immediate environment. Maintain patient in private room or >3 feet away from other patients.
Droplet	Use mask while caring for the patient. Maintain patient in a private room or >3 feet away from other patients with curtain separating them. Use patient mask if transporting patient from one area to another.
Airborne	Place patient in an airborne infection isolation room. Use ≥N95 respirators (or masks) while caring for patient.

43. D: Chemical debridement is used for chronic wounds (burns, ulcers) with necrotic tissue and eschar. However the enzymes (collagenase and papain/urea) require a moist environment, so the eschar must be cross-hatched through the upper layers before the enzyme is administered. The pH must remain between 6 and 8 to prevent inactivation. Hexachlorophene, Burrow's solution, and heavy metal ions also inactivate the enzymes. Collagenase is applied one time daily, either directly to the wound for deep wounds or to gauze packing for shallow wounds.

44. A: These VS changes are consistent with increasing intracranial pressure. Typical findings include widened pulse pressure, with rising blood pressure and depressed heart rate. Because the patient is drunk, evaluating level of consciousness can be difficult, but lethargy, confusion, and restlessness are characteristic of increasing ICP. Stress response usually results in increased BP and pulse. Ethanol intoxication usually causes hypotension, bradycardia with arrhythmias, and respiratory depression. Delirium tremens includes tremors, tachycardia, and cardiac dysrhythmias.

45. B: "Patient is spitting at nurses, throwing magazines, and refusing to get out of bed for therapy" describes the patient's behavior without placing a value judgment ("belligerent and uncooperative"), which might indicate bias against the patient. The nurse should avoid interpreting behavior ("appears to dislike") or characterizing what's in a patient's mind ("Patient believes"). Patients, especially older adults or those who are confused, may behave in a difficult manner if they are afraid, in pain, or overwhelmed, so the nurse should attempt to find the reason for the behavior.

46. A: St. John's wort may interact with antibiotics, birth control pills, antidepressants, warfarin, anticonvulsants, MAO inhibitors, antivirals, immunosuppressants, and migraine drugs. Melatonin may interact with NSAIDS, antihypertensives, steroids, and anti-anxiety medications. Echinacea may interact with immunosuppressants and steroids. Vitamin B complex is safe to take with warfarin, as it does not affect the INR; however, multivitamins with vitamin K may. If patients take a multivitamin during warfarin therapy, they should do so daily and not intermittently so that intake of vitamin K does not fluctuate. Vitamin C should be limited to 500 mg daily and vitamin E to 400 IU daily.

47. D: Root cause analysis is a retrospective attempt to determine the cause of an event. Regression analysis compares the relationship between two variables to determine if the relationship correlates. T-test is used to analyze data to determine if there is a statistically

significant difference in the means of two groups. The t-test looks at two sets of things that are similar, such as exercise in women over 65 with cancer and over 65 without cancer. Tracer methodology is a method that looks at the continuum of care a patient receives from admission to post-discharge.

48. D: The best solution is a referral to a home health agency to provide in-home care, as this ensures that the woman will receive skilled nursing care and be able to stay at home and supervise her granddaughter. A 12-year-old is too young for the responsibility of wound care. The patient's dependence on public transportation and difficulty walking precludes outpatient care. Home health care is a more cost-effective solution than transferring the patient to an extended care facility, which would leave the granddaughter without care. Medicare will not pay for extended hospital care for healing wounds.

49. B: This is an example of selection bias because those with catheters without clinically evident infections were excluded. The results are skewed because many patients may have subclinical infections. Information bias occurs when there are errors in classification, so an estimate of association is incorrect. Information bias may be non-differential or differential. Compliance bias occurs when adherence to protocol is inconsistent. Admission bias occurs when some groups, such as spinal cord injury patients, are omitted from the study.

50. D: These symptoms are consistent with pacemaker syndrome.

Mild	Pulsations evident in neck and abdomen. Cardiac palpitations. Headache and feeling of anxiety. General malaise and unexplained weakness. Pain or "fullness" in jaw, chest.
Moderate	Increasing dyspnea on exertion with accompanying orthopnea Dizziness, vertigo, increasing confusion. Feeling of choking.
Severe	Increasing pulmonary edema with dyspnea even at rest and crackling rales. Syncope. Heart failure.

Secret Key #1 - Time is Your Greatest Enemy

Pace Yourself

Wear a watch. At the beginning of the test, check the time (or start a chronometer on your watch to count the minutes), and check the time after every few questions to make sure you are "on schedule."

If you are forced to speed up, do it efficiently. Usually one or more answer choices can be eliminated without too much difficulty. Above all, don't panic. Don't speed up and just begin guessing at random choices. By pacing yourself, and continually monitoring your progress against your watch, you will always know exactly how far ahead or behind you are with your available time. If you find that you are one minute behind on the test, don't skip one question without spending any time on it, just to catch back up. Take 15 fewer seconds on the next four questions, and after four questions you'll have caught back up. Once you catch back up, you can continue working each problem at your normal pace.

Furthermore, don't dwell on the problems that you were rushed on. If a problem was taking up too much time and you made a hurried guess, it must be difficult. The difficult questions are the ones you are most likely to miss anyway, so it isn't a big loss. It is better to end with more time than you need than to run out of time.

Lastly, sometimes it is beneficial to slow down if you are constantly getting ahead of time. You are always more likely to catch a careless mistake by working more slowly than quickly, and among very high-scoring test takers (those who are likely to have lots of time left over), careless errors affect the score more than mastery of material.

Secret Key #2 - Guessing is not Guesswork

You probably know that guessing is a good idea. Unlike other standardized tests, there is no penalty for getting a wrong answer. Even if you have no idea about a question, you still have a 20-25% chance of getting it right.

Most test takers do not understand the impact that proper guessing can have on their score. Unless you score extremely high, guessing will significantly contribute to your final score.

Monkeys Take the Test

What most test takers don't realize is that to insure that 20-25% chance, you have to guess randomly. If you put 20 monkeys in a room to take this test, assuming they answered once per question and behaved themselves, on average they would get 20-25% of the questions correct. Put 20 test takers in the room, and the average will be much lower among guessed questions. Why?
  1. The test writers intentionally write deceptive answer choices that "look" right. A test

taker has no idea about a question, so he picks the "best looking" answer, which is often wrong. The monkey has no idea what looks good and what doesn't, so it will consistently be right about 20-25% of the time.

2. Test takers will eliminate answer choices from the guessing pool based on a hunch or intuition. Simple but correct answers often get excluded, leaving a 0% chance of being correct. The monkey has no clue, and often gets lucky with the best choice.

This is why the process of elimination endorsed by most test courses is flawed and detrimental to your performance. Test takers don't guess; they make an ignorant stab in the dark that is usually worse than random.

$5 Challenge

Let me introduce one of the most valuable ideas of this course—the $5 challenge:

You only mark your "best guess" if you are willing to bet $5 on it.
You only eliminate choices from guessing if you are willing to bet $5 on it.

Why $5? Five dollars is an amount of money that is small yet not insignificant, and can really add up fast (20 questions could cost you $100). Likewise, each answer choice on one question of the test will have a small impact on your overall score, but it can really add up to a lot of points in the end.

The process of elimination IS valuable. The following shows your chance of guessing it right:

If you eliminate wrong answer choices until only this many remain:	Chance of getting it correct:
1	100%
2	50%
3	33%

However, if you accidentally eliminate the right answer or go on a hunch for an incorrect answer, your chances drop dramatically—to 0%. By guessing among all the answer choices, you are GUARANTEED to have a shot at the right answer.

That's why the $5 test is so valuable. If you give up the advantage and safety of a pure guess, it had better be worth the risk.

What we still haven't covered is how to be sure that whatever guess you make is truly random. Here's the easiest way:

Always pick the first answer choice among those remaining.

Such a technique means that you have decided, **before you see a single test question**, exactly how you are going to guess, and since the order of choices tells you nothing about which one is correct, this guessing technique is perfectly random.

This section is not meant to scare you away from making educated guesses or eliminating choices; you just need to define when a choice is worth eliminating. The $5 test, along with a pre-defined random guessing strategy, is the best way to make sure you reap all of the benefits of guessing.

Secret Key #3 - Practice Smarter, Not Harder

Many test takers delay the test preparation process because they dread the awful amounts of practice time they think necessary to succeed on the test. We have refined an effective method that will take you only a fraction of the time.

There are a number of "obstacles" in the path to success. Among these are answering questions, finishing in time, and mastering test-taking strategies. All must be executed on the day of the test at peak performance, or your score will suffer. The test is a mental marathon that has a large impact on your future.

Just like a marathon runner, it is important to work your way up to the full challenge. So first you just worry about questions, and then time, and finally strategy:

Success Strategy

1. Find a good source for practice tests.
2. If you are willing to make a larger time investment, consider using more than one study guide. Often the different approaches of multiple authors will help you "get" difficult concepts.
3. Take a practice test with no time constraints, with all study helps, "open book." Take your time with questions and focus on applying strategies.
4. Take a practice test with time constraints, with all guides, "open book."
5. Take a final practice test without open material and with time limits.

If you have time to take more practice tests, just repeat step 5. By gradually exposing yourself to the full rigors of the test environment, you will condition your mind to the stress of test day and maximize your success.

Secret Key #4 - Prepare, Don't Procrastinate

Let me state an obvious fact: if you take the test three times, you will probably get three different scores. This is due to the way you feel on test day, the level of preparedness you have, and the version of the test you see. Despite the test writers' claims to the contrary, some versions of the test WILL be easier for you than others.

Since your future depends so much on your score, you should maximize your chances of success. In order to maximize the likelihood of success, you've got to prepare in advance.

This means taking practice tests and spending time learning the information and test taking strategies you will need to succeed.

Never go take the actual test as a "practice" test, expecting that you can just take it again if you need to. Take all the practice tests you can on your own, but when you go to take the official test, be prepared, be focused, and do your best the first time!

Secret Key #5 - Test Yourself

Everyone knows that time is money. There is no need to spend too much of your time or too little of your time preparing for the test. You should only spend as much of your precious time preparing as is necessary for you to get the score you need.

Once you have taken a practice test under real conditions of time constraints, then you will know if you are ready for the test or not.

If you have scored extremely high the first time that you take the practice test, then there is not much point in spending countless hours studying. You are already there.

Benchmark your abilities by retaking practice tests and seeing how much you have improved. Once you consistently score high enough to guarantee success, then you are ready.

If you have scored well below where you need, then knuckle down and begin studying in earnest. Check your improvement regularly through the use of practice tests under real conditions. Above all, don't worry, panic, or give up. The key is perseverance!

Then, when you go to take the test, remain confident and remember how well you did on the practice tests. If you can score high enough on a practice test, then you can do the same on the real thing.

General Strategies

The most important thing you can do is to ignore your fears and jump into the test immediately. Do not be overwhelmed by any strange-sounding terms. You have to jump into the test like jumping into a pool—all at once is the easiest way.

Make Predictions

As you read and understand the question, try to guess what the answer will be. Remember that several of the answer choices are wrong, and once you begin reading them, your mind will immediately become cluttered with answer choices designed to throw you off. Your mind is typically the most focused immediately after you have read the question and digested its contents. If you can, try to predict what the correct answer will be. You may be surprised at what you can predict.

Quickly scan the choices and see if your prediction is in the listed answer choices. If it is, then you can be quite confident that you have the right answer. It still won't hurt to check the other answer choices, but most of the time, you've got it!

Answer the Question

It may seem obvious to only pick answer choices that answer the question, but the test writers can create some excellent answer choices that are wrong. Don't pick an answer just because it sounds right, or you believe it to be true. It MUST answer the question. Once you've made your selection, always go back and check it against the question and make sure that you didn't misread the question and that the answer choice does answer the question posed.

Benchmark

After you read the first answer choice, decide if you think it sounds correct or not. If it doesn't, move on to the next answer choice. If it does, mentally mark that answer choice. This doesn't mean that you've definitely selected it as your answer choice, it just means that it's the best you've seen thus far. Go ahead and read the next choice. If the next choice is worse than the one you've already selected, keep going to the next answer choice. If the next choice is better than the choice you've already selected, mentally mark the new answer choice as your best guess.

The first answer choice that you select becomes your standard. Every other answer choice must be benchmarked against that standard. That choice is correct until proven otherwise by another answer choice beating it out. Once you've decided that no other answer choice seems as good, do one final check to ensure that your answer choice answers the question posed.

Valid Information

Don't discount any of the information provided in the question. Every piece of information may be necessary to determine the correct answer. None of the information in the question is there to throw you off (while the answer choices will certainly have information to throw you off). If two seemingly unrelated topics are discussed, don't ignore either. You can be confident there is a relationship, or it wouldn't be included in the question, and you are probably going to have to determine what is that relationship to find the answer.

Avoid "Fact Traps"

Don't get distracted by a choice that is factually true. Your search is for the answer that answers the question. Stay focused and don't fall for an answer that is true but irrelevant. Always go back to the question and make sure you're choosing an answer that actually answers the question and is not just a true statement. An answer can be factually correct, but it MUST answer the question asked. Additionally, two answers can both be seemingly correct, so be sure to read all of the answer choices, and make sure that you get the one that BEST answers the question.

Milk the Question

Some of the questions may throw you completely off. They might deal with a subject you have not been exposed to, or one that you haven't reviewed in years. While your lack of knowledge about the subject will be a hindrance, the question itself can give you many clues that will help you find the correct answer. Read the question carefully and look for clues. Watch particularly for adjectives and nouns describing difficult terms or words that you

- 136 -

don't recognize. Regardless of whether you completely understand a word or not, replacing it with a synonym, either provided or one you more familiar with, may help you to understand what the questions are asking. Rather than wracking your mind about specific detailed information concerning a difficult term or word, try to use mental substitutes that are easier to understand.

The Trap of Familiarity

Don't just choose a word because you recognize it. On difficult questions, you may not recognize a number of words in the answer choices. The test writers don't put "make-believe" words on the test, so don't think that just because you only recognize all the words in one answer choice that that answer choice must be correct. If you only recognize words in one answer choice, then focus on that one. Is it correct? Try your best to determine if it is correct. If it is, that's great. If not, eliminate it. Each word and answer choice you eliminate increases your chances of getting the question correct, even if you then have to guess among the unfamiliar choices.

Eliminate Answers

Eliminate choices as soon as you realize they are wrong. But be careful! Make sure you consider all of the possible answer choices. Just because one appears right, doesn't mean that the next one won't be even better! The test writers will usually put more than one good answer choice for every question, so read all of them. Don't worry if you are stuck between two that seem right. By getting down to just two remaining possible choices, your odds are now 50/50. Rather than wasting too much time, play the odds. You are guessing, but guessing wisely because you've been able to knock out some of the answer choices that you know are wrong. If you are eliminating choices and realize that the last answer choice you are left with is also obviously wrong, don't panic. Start over and consider each choice again. There may easily be something that you missed the first time and will realize on the second pass.

Tough Questions

If you are stumped on a problem or it appears too hard or too difficult, don't waste time. Move on! Remember though, if you can quickly check for obviously incorrect answer choices, your chances of guessing correctly are greatly improved. Before you completely give up, at least try to knock out a couple of possible answers. Eliminate what you can and then guess at the remaining answer choices before moving on.

Brainstorm

If you get stuck on a difficult question, spend a few seconds quickly brainstorming. Run through the complete list of possible answer choices. Look at each choice and ask yourself, "Could this answer the question satisfactorily?" Go through each answer choice and consider it independently of the others. By systematically going through all possibilities, you may find something that you would otherwise overlook. Remember though that when you get stuck, it's important to try to keep moving.

Read Carefully

Understand the problem. Read the question and answer choices carefully. Don't miss the question because you misread the terms. You have plenty of time to read each question thoroughly and make sure you understand what is being asked. Yet a happy medium must be attained, so don't waste too much time. You must read carefully, but efficiently.

Face Value

When in doubt, use common sense. Always accept the situation in the problem at face value. Don't read too much into it. These problems will not require you to make huge leaps of logic. The test writers aren't trying to throw you off with a cheap trick. If you have to go beyond creativity and make a leap of logic in order to have an answer choice answer the question, then you should look at the other answer choices. Don't overcomplicate the problem by creating theoretical relationships or explanations that will warp time or space. These are normal problems rooted in reality. It's just that the applicable relationship or explanation may not be readily apparent and you have to figure things out. Use your common sense to interpret anything that isn't clear.

Prefixes

If you're having trouble with a word in the question or answer choices, try dissecting it. Take advantage of every clue that the word might include. Prefixes and suffixes can be a huge help. Usually they allow you to determine a basic meaning. Pre- means before, post- means after, pro - is positive, de- is negative. From these prefixes and suffixes, you can get an idea of the general meaning of the word and try to put it into context. Beware though of any traps. Just because con- is the opposite of pro-, doesn't necessarily mean congress is the opposite of progress!

Hedge Phrases

Watch out for critical hedge phrases, led off with words such as "likely," "may," "can," "sometimes," "often," "almost," "mostly," "usually," "generally," "rarely," and "sometimes." Question writers insert these hedge phrases to cover every possibility. Often an answer choice will be wrong simply because it leaves no room for exception. Unless the situation calls for them, avoid answer choices that have definitive words like "exactly," and "always."

Switchback Words

Stay alert for "switchbacks." These are the words and phrases frequently used to alert you to shifts in thought. The most common switchback word is "but." Others include "although," "however," "nevertheless," "on the other hand," "even though," "while," "in spite of," "despite," and "regardless of."

New Information

Correct answer choices will rarely have completely new information included. Answer choices typically are straightforward reflections of the material asked about and will directly relate to the question. If a new piece of information is included in an answer choice that doesn't even seem to relate to the topic being asked about, then that answer choice is likely incorrect. All of the information needed to answer the question is usually provided for you in the question. You should not have to make guesses that are unsupported or choose answer choices that require unknown information that cannot be reasoned from what is given.

Time Management

On technical questions, don't get lost on the technical terms. Don't spend too much time on any one question. If you don't know what a term means, then odds are you aren't going to get much further since you don't have a dictionary. You should be able to immediately recognize whether or not you know a term. If you don't, work with the other clues that you have—the other answer choices and terms provided—but don't waste too much time trying to figure out a difficult term that you don't know.

Contextual Clues

Look for contextual clues. An answer can be right but not the correct answer. The contextual clues will help you find the answer that is most right and is correct. Understand the context in which a phrase or statement is made. This will help you make important distinctions.

Don't Panic

Panicking will not answer any questions for you; therefore, it isn't helpful. When you first see the question, if your mind goes blank, take a deep breath. Force yourself to mechanically go through the steps of solving the problem using the strategies you've learned.

Pace Yourself

Don't get clock fever. It's easy to be overwhelmed when you're looking at a page full of questions, your mind is full of random thoughts and feeling confused, and the clock is ticking down faster than you would like. Calm down and maintain the pace that you have set for yourself. As long as you are on track by monitoring your pace, you are guaranteed to have enough time for yourself. When you get to the last few minutes of the test, it may seem like you won't have enough time left, but if you only have as many questions as you should have left at that point, then you're right on track!

Answer Selection

The best way to pick an answer choice is to eliminate all of those that are wrong, until only one is left and confirm that is the correct answer. Sometimes though, an answer choice may immediately look right. Be careful! Take a second to make sure that the other choices are not equally obvious. Don't make a hasty mistake. There are only two times that you should stop before checking other answers. First is when you are positive that the answer choice you have selected is correct. Second is when time is almost out and you have to make a quick guess!

Check Your Work

Since you will probably not know every term listed and the answer to every question, it is important that you get credit for the ones that you do know. Don't miss any questions through careless mistakes. If at all possible, try to take a second to look back over your answer selection and make sure you've selected the correct answer choice and haven't made a costly careless mistake (such as marking an answer choice that you didn't mean to mark). The time it takes for this quick double check should more than pay for itself in caught mistakes.

Beware of Directly Quoted Answers

Sometimes an answer choice will repeat word for word a portion of the question or reference section. However, beware of such exact duplication. It may be a trap! More than likely, the correct choice will paraphrase or summarize a point, rather than being exactly the same wording.

Slang

Scientific sounding answers are better than slang ones. An answer choice that begins "To compare the outcomes…" is much more likely to be correct than one that begins "Because some people insisted…"

Extreme Statements

Avoid wild answers that throw out highly controversial ideas that are proclaimed as established fact. An answer choice that states the "process should used in certain situations, if…" is much more likely to be correct than one that states the "process should be discontinued completely." The first is a calm rational statement and doesn't even make a definitive, uncompromising stance, using a hedge word "if" to provide wiggle room, whereas the second choice is a radical idea and far more extreme.

Answer Choice Families

When you have two or more answer choices that are direct opposites or parallels, one of them is usually the correct answer. For instance, if one answer choice states "x increases" and another answer choice states "x decreases" or "y increases," then those two or three answer choices are very similar in construction and fall into the same family of answer choices. A family of answer choices consists of two or three answer choices, very similar in construction, but often with directly opposite meanings. Usually the correct answer choice will be in that family of answer choices. The "odd man out" or answer choice that doesn't seem to fit the parallel construction of the other answer choices is more likely to be incorrect.

Special Report: How to Overcome Test Anxiety

The very nature of tests caters to some level of anxiety, nervousness, or tension, just as we feel for any important event that occurs in our lives. A little bit of anxiety or nervousness can be a good thing. It helps us with motivation, and makes achievement just that much sweeter. However, too much anxiety can be a problem, especially if it hinders our ability to function and perform.

"Test anxiety," is the term that refers to the emotional reactions that some test-takers experience when faced with a test or exam. Having a fear of testing and exams is based upon a rational fear, since the test-taker's performance can shape the course of an academic career. Nevertheless, experiencing excessive fear of examinations will only interfere with the test-taker's ability to perform and chance to be successful.

There are a large variety of causes that can contribute to the development and sensation of test anxiety. These include, but are not limited to, lack of preparation and worrying about issues surrounding the test.

Lack of Preparation

Lack of preparation can be identified by the following behaviors or situations:

Not scheduling enough time to study, and therefore cramming the night before the test or exam
Managing time poorly, to create the sensation that there is not enough time to do everything
Failing to organize the text information in advance, so that the study material consists of the entire text and not simply the pertinent information
Poor overall studying habits

Worrying, on the other hand, can be related to both the test taker, or many other factors around him/her that will be affected by the results of the test. These include worrying about:

Previous performances on similar exams, or exams in general
How friends and other students are achieving
The negative consequences that will result from a poor grade or failure

There are three primary elements to test anxiety. Physical components, which involve the same typical bodily reactions as those to acute anxiety (to be discussed below). Emotional factors have to do with fear or panic. Mental or cognitive issues concerning attention spans and memory abilities.

Physical Signals

There are many different symptoms of test anxiety, and these are not limited to mental and emotional strain. Frequently there are a range of physical signals that will let a test taker know that he/she is suffering from test anxiety. These bodily changes can include the following:

Perspiring
Sweaty palms
Wet, trembling hands
Nausea
Dry mouth
A knot in the stomach
Headache
Faintness
Muscle tension
Aching shoulders, back and neck
Rapid heart beat
Feeling too hot/cold

To recognize the sensation of test anxiety, a test-taker should monitor him/herself for the following sensations:

The physical distress symptoms as listed above
Emotional sensitivity, expressing emotional feelings such as the need to cry or laugh too much, or a sensation of anger or helplessness
A decreased ability to think, causing the test-taker to blank out or have racing thoughts that are hard to organize or control.

Though most students will feel some level of anxiety when faced with a test or exam, the majority can cope with that anxiety and maintain it at a manageable level. However, those who cannot are faced with a very real and very serious condition, which can and should be controlled for the immeasurable benefit of this sufferer.

Naturally, these sensations lead to negative results for the testing experience. The most common effects of test anxiety have to do with nervousness and mental blocking.

Nervousness

Nervousness can appear in several different levels:

The test-taker's difficulty, or even inability to read and understand the questions on the test
The difficulty or inability to organize thoughts to a coherent form
The difficulty or inability to recall key words and concepts relating to the testing questions (especially essays)
The receipt of poor grades on a test, though the test material was well known by the test taker

Conversely, a person may also experience mental blocking, which involves:

Blanking out on test questions
Only remembering the correct answers to the questions when the test has already finished.

Fortunately for test anxiety sufferers, beating these feelings, to a large degree, has to do with proper preparation. When a test taker has a feeling of preparedness, then anxiety will be dramatically lessened.

The first step to resolving anxiety issues is to distinguish which of the two types of anxiety are being suffered. If the anxiety is a direct result of a lack of preparation, this should be considered a normal reaction, and the anxiety level (as opposed to the test results) shouldn't be anything to worry about. However, if, when adequately prepared, the test-taker still panics, blanks out, or seems to overreact, this is not a fully rational reaction. While this can be considered normal too, there are many ways to combat and overcome these effects.

Remember that anxiety cannot be entirely eliminated, however, there are ways to minimize it, to make the anxiety easier to manage. Preparation is one of the best ways to minimize test anxiety. Therefore the following techniques are wise in order to best fight off any anxiety that may want to build.

To begin with, try to avoid cramming before a test, whenever it is possible. By trying to memorize an entire term's worth of information in one day, you'll be shocking your system, and not giving yourself a very good chance to absorb the information. This is an easy path to anxiety, so for those who suffer from test anxiety, cramming should not even be considered an option.

Instead of cramming, work throughout the semester to combine all of the material which is presented throughout the semester, and work on it gradually as the course goes by, making sure to master the main concepts first, leaving minor details for a week or so before the test.

To study for the upcoming exam, be sure to pose questions that may be on the examination, to gauge the ability to answer them by integrating the ideas from your texts, notes and lectures, as well as any supplementary readings.

If it is truly impossible to cover all of the information that was covered in that particular term, concentrate on the most important portions, that can be covered very well. Learn these concepts as best as possible, so that when the test comes, a goal can be made to use these concepts as presentations of your knowledge.

In addition to study habits, changes in attitude are critical to beating a struggle with test anxiety. In fact, an improvement of the perspective over the entire test-taking experience can actually help a test taker to enjoy studying and therefore improve the overall experience. Be certain not to overemphasize the significance of the grade - know that the result of the test is neither a reflection of self worth, nor is it a measure of intelligence; one grade will not predict a person's future success.

To improve an overall testing outlook, the following steps should be tried:

Keeping in mind that the most reasonable expectation for taking a test is to expect to try to demonstrate as much of what you know as you possibly can.
Reminding ourselves that a test is only one test; this is not the only one, and there will be others.
The thought of thinking of oneself in an irrational, all-or-nothing term should be avoided at all costs.
A reward should be designated for after the test, so there's something to look forward to. Whether it be going to a movie, going out to eat, or simply visiting friends, schedule it in advance, and do it no matter what result is expected on the exam.

Test-takers should also keep in mind that the basics are some of the most important things, even beyond anti-anxiety techniques and studying. Never neglect the basic social, emotional and biological needs, in order to try to absorb information. In order to best achieve, these three factors must be held as just as important as the studying itself.

Study Steps

Remember the following important steps for studying:

Maintain healthy nutrition and exercise habits. Continue both your recreational activities and social pass times. These both contribute to your physical and emotional well being.
Be certain to get a good amount of sleep, especially the night before the test, because when you're overtired you are not able to perform to the best of your best ability.
Keep the studying pace to a moderate level by taking breaks when they are needed, and varying the work whenever possible, to keep the mind fresh instead of getting bored. When enough studying has been done that all the material that can be learned has been learned, and the test taker is prepared for the test, stop studying and do something relaxing such as listening to music, watching a movie, or taking a warm bubble bath.

There are also many other techniques to minimize the uneasiness or apprehension that is experienced along with test anxiety before, during, or even after the examination. In fact, there are a great deal of things that can be done to stop anxiety from interfering with lifestyle and performance. Again, remember that anxiety will not be eliminated entirely, and it shouldn't be. Otherwise that "up" feeling for exams would not exist, and most of us depend on that sensation to perform better than usual. However, this anxiety has to be at a level that is manageable.

Of course, as we have just discussed, being prepared for the exam is half the battle right away. Attending all classes, finding out what knowledge will be expected on the exam, and knowing the exam schedules are easy steps to lowering anxiety. Keeping up with work will remove the need to cram, and efficient study habits will eliminate wasted time. Studying should be done in an ideal location for concentration, so that it is simple to become interested in the material and give it complete attention. A method such as SQ3R (Survey, Question, Read, Recite, Review) is a wonderful key to follow to make sure that the study habits are as effective as possible, especially in the case of learning from a textbook. Flashcards are great techniques for memorization. Learning to take good notes will mean that notes will be full of useful information, so that less sifting will need to be done to seek out what is pertinent for studying. Reviewing notes after class and then again on occasion will keep the information fresh in the mind. From notes that have been taken summary sheets and outlines can be made for simpler reviewing.

A study group can also be a very motivational and helpful place to study, as there will be a sharing of ideas, all of the minds can work together, to make sure that everyone understands, and the studying will be made more interesting because it will be a social occasion.

Basically, though, as long as the test-taker remains organized and self confident, with efficient study habits, less time will need to be spent studying, and higher grades will be achieved.

To become self confident, there are many useful steps. The first of these is "self talk." It has been shown through extensive research, that self-talk for students who suffer from test anxiety, should be well monitored, in order to make sure that it contributes to self confidence as opposed to sinking the student. Frequently the self talk of test-anxious students is negative or self-defeating, thinking that everyone else is smarter and faster, that they always mess up, and that if they don't do well, they'll fail the entire course. It is important to decreasing anxiety that awareness is made of self talk. Try writing any negative self thoughts and then disputing them with a positive statement instead. Begin self-encouragement as though it was a friend speaking. Repeat positive statements to help reprogram the mind to believing in successes instead of failures.

Helpful Techniques

Other extremely helpful techniques include:

Self-visualization of doing well and reaching goals
While aiming for an "A" level of understanding, don't try to "overprotect" by setting your expectations lower. This will only convince the mind to stop studying in order to meet the lower expectations.
Don't make comparisons with the results or habits of other students. These are individual factors, and different things work for different people, causing different results.
Strive to become an expert in learning what works well, and what can be done in order to improve. Consider collecting this data in a journal.
Create rewards for after studying instead of doing things before studying that will only turn into avoidance behaviors.
Make a practice of relaxing - by using methods such as progressive relaxation, self-hypnosis, guided imagery, etc - in order to make relaxation an automatic sensation.
Work on creating a state of relaxed concentration so that concentrating will take on the focus of the mind, so that none will be wasted on worrying.
Take good care of the physical self by eating well and getting enough sleep.
Plan in time for exercise and stick to this plan.

Beyond these techniques, there are other methods to be used before, during and after the test that will help the test-taker perform well in addition to overcoming anxiety.

Before the exam comes the academic preparation. This involves establishing a study schedule and beginning at least one week before the actual date of the test. By doing this, the anxiety of not having enough time to study for the test will be automatically eliminated. Moreover, this will make the studying a much more effective experience, ensuring that the learning will be an easier process. This relieves much undue pressure on the test-taker.

Summary sheets, note cards, and flash cards with the main concepts and examples of these main concepts should be prepared in advance of the actual studying time. A topic should never be eliminated from this process. By omitting a topic because it isn't expected to be on the test is only setting up the test-taker for anxiety should it actually appear on the exam. Utilize the course syllabus for laying out the topics that should be studied. Carefully go over the notes that were made in class, paying special attention to any of the issues that the professor took special care to emphasize while lecturing in class. In the textbooks, use the chapter review, or if possible, the chapter tests, to begin your review.

It may even be possible to ask the instructor what information will be covered on the exam, or what the format of the exam will be (for example, multiple choice, essay, free form, true-false). Additionally, see if it is possible to find out how many questions will be on the test. If a review sheet or sample test has been offered by the professor, make good use of it, above anything else, for the preparation for the test. Another great resource for getting to know the examination is reviewing tests from previous semesters. Use these tests to review, and aim to achieve a 100% score on each of the possible topics. With a few exceptions, the goal that you set for yourself is the highest one that you will reach.

Take all of the questions that were assigned as homework, and rework them to any other possible course material. The more problems reworked, the more skill and confidence will form as a result. When forming the solution to a problem, write out each of the steps. Don't simply do head work. By doing as many steps on paper as possible, much clarification and therefore confidence will be formed. Do this with as many homework problems as possible, before checking the answers. By checking the answer after each problem, a reinforcement will exist, that will not be on the exam. Study situations should be as exam-like as possible, to prime the test-taker's system for the experience. By waiting to check the answers at the end, a psychological advantage will be formed, to decrease the stress factor.

Another fantastic reason for not cramming is the avoidance of confusion in concepts, especially when it comes to mathematics. 8-10 hours of study will become one hundred percent more effective if it is spread out over a week or at least several days, instead of doing it all in one sitting. Recognize that the human brain requires time in order to assimilate new material, so frequent breaks and a span of study time over several days will be much more beneficial.

Additionally, don't study right up until the point of the exam. Studying should stop a minimum of one hour before the exam begins. This allows the brain to rest and put things in their proper order. This will also provide the time to become as relaxed as possible when going into the examination room. The test-taker will also have time to eat well and eat sensibly. Know that the brain needs food as much as the rest of the body. With enough food and enough sleep, as well as a relaxed attitude, the body and the mind are primed for success.

Avoid any anxious classmates who are talking about the exam. These students only spread anxiety, and are not worth sharing the anxious sentimentalities.

Before the test also involves creating a positive attitude, so mental preparation should also be a point of concentration. There are many keys to creating a positive attitude. Should fears become rushing in, make a visualization of taking the exam, doing well, and seeing an A written on the paper. Write out a list of affirmations that will bring a feeling of confidence, such as "I am doing well in my English class," "I studied well and know my material," "I enjoy this class." Even if the affirmations aren't believed at first, it sends a positive message to the subconscious which will result in an alteration of the overall belief system, which is the system that creates reality.

If a sensation of panic begins, work with the fear and imagine the very worst! Work through the entire scenario of not passing the test, failing the entire course, and dropping out of school, followed by not getting a job, and pushing a shopping cart through the dark alley where you'll live. This will place things into perspective! Then, practice deep breathing and create a visualization of the opposite situation - achieving an "A" on the exam, passing the entire course, receiving the degree at a graduation ceremony.

On the day of the test, there are many things to be done to ensure the best results, as well as the most calm outlook. The following stages are suggested in order to maximize test-taking potential:

Begin the examination day with a moderate breakfast, and avoid any coffee or beverages with caffeine if the test taker is prone to jitters. Even people who are used to managing caffeine can feel jittery or light-headed when it is taken on a test day.
Attempt to do something that is relaxing before the examination begins. As last minute cramming clouds the mastering of overall concepts, it is better to use this time to create a calming outlook.
Be certain to arrive at the test location well in advance, in order to provide time to select a location that is away from doors, windows and other distractions, as well as giving enough time to relax before the test begins.
Keep away from anxiety generating classmates who will upset the sensation of stability and relaxation that is being attempted before the exam.
Should the waiting period before the exam begins cause anxiety, create a self-distraction by reading a light magazine or something else that is relaxing and simple.

During the exam itself, read the entire exam from beginning to end, and find out how much time should be allotted to each individual problem. Once writing the exam, should more time be taken for a problem, it should be abandoned, in order to begin another problem. If there is time at the end, the unfinished problem can always be returned to and completed.

Read the instructions very carefully - twice - so that unpleasant surprises won't follow during or after the exam has ended.

When writing the exam, pretend that the situation is actually simply the completion of homework within a library, or at home. This will assist in forming a relaxed atmosphere, and will allow the brain extra focus for the complex thinking function.

Begin the exam with all of the questions with which the most confidence is felt. This will build the confidence level regarding the entire exam and will begin a quality momentum. This will also create encouragement for trying the problems where uncertainty resides.

Going with the "gut instinct" is always the way to go when solving a problem. Second guessing should be avoided at all costs. Have confidence in the ability to do well.

For essay questions, create an outline in advance that will keep the mind organized and make certain that all of the points are remembered. For multiple choice, read every answer, even if the correct one has been spotted - a better one may exist.

Continue at a pace that is reasonable and not rushed, in order to be able to work carefully. Provide enough time to go over the answers at the end, to check for small errors that can be corrected.

Should a feeling of panic begin, breathe deeply, and think of the feeling of the body releasing sand through its pores. Visualize a calm, peaceful place, and include all of the sights, sounds and sensations of this image. Continue the deep breathing, and take a few minutes to continue this with closed eyes. When all is well again, return to the test.

If a "blanking" occurs for a certain question, skip it and move on to the next question. There will be time to return to the other question later. Get everything done that can be done, first, to guarantee all the grades that can be compiled, and to build all of the confidence possible. Then return to the weaker questions to build the marks from there.

Remember, one's own reality can be created, so as long as the belief is there, success will follow. And remember: anxiety can happen later, right now, there's an exam to be written!

After the examination is complete, whether there is a feeling for a good grade or a bad grade, don't dwell on the exam, and be certain to follow through on the reward that was promised...and enjoy it! Don't dwell on any mistakes that have been made, as there is nothing that can be done at this point anyway.

Additionally, don't begin to study for the next test right away. Do something relaxing for a while, and let the mind relax and prepare itself to begin absorbing information again.

From the results of the exam - both the grade and the entire experience, be certain to learn from what has gone on. Perfect studying habits and work some more on confidence in order to make the next examination experience even better than the last one.

Learn to avoid places where openings occurred for laziness, procrastination and day dreaming.

Use the time between this exam and the next one to better learn to relax, even learning to relax on cue, so that any anxiety can be controlled during the next exam. Learn how to relax the body. Slouch in your chair if that helps. Tighten and then relax all of the different muscle groups, one group at a time, beginning with the feet and then working all the way up to the neck and face. This will ultimately relax the muscles more than they were to begin with. Learn how to breathe deeply and comfortably, and focus on this breathing going in and out as a relaxing thought. With every exhale, repeat the word "relax."

As common as test anxiety is, it is very possible to overcome it. Make yourself one of the test-takers who overcome this frustrating hindrance.

Special Report: Additional Bonus Material

Due to our efforts to try to keep this book to a manageable length, we've created a link that will give you access to all of your additional bonus material.

Please visit http://www.mometrix.com/bonus948/npadgeracutec to access the information.